Role of Proteomics in High Altitude Pathophysiology

Yasmin Ahmad
Aditya Arya

Published by iConcept Press Limited

Published by iConcept Press Limited

Copyright © iConcept Press 2016

http://www.iconceptpress.com

ISBN: 978-1-922227-553

Printed in the United States of America

Contents

Preface

High altitude physiology is one of the ignored domain of the scientific research despite of the massive scale of the problem, suggested by nearly 24% of the global population that either visits or dwells at high altitude and remain at the risk of hypoxia associated alterations in physiology. This lecture note entitled "Role of Proteomics in High altitude Pathophysiology" is designed especially for those who are interested in learning proteomics and their application in the field of high altitude physiology. It meets the needs of the proteomics studies prescribed for the high altitude physiology as it covers pathophysiology and molecular biology of high altitude sickness, proteomics as powerful tools and major proteomic advancements on pathophysiology of acute mountain sickness.

This lecture notes has 5 units and can be completed in two sessions. Initially, we introduced the term hypobaric hypoxia as a socio-economic problem followed by the description of its pathophysiology. The later chapters describe the role of proteomics and key findings of our lab. Finally a last concluding chapter includes the future guidelines for improving the health benefits of the ongoing research and developing novel strategies for future research. Though this lecture note has been designed for the students of biology field, it would be useful also for clinical professionals in the early stage of their career. It would be helpful to anyone who desires to enhance their knowledge in the field of high altitude physiology.

Yasmin Ahmad and Aditya Arya

1

Introduction

Hypoxia causes a sequence of physiologic changes that help the body to adapt or acclimatize to the conditions. Successful acclimatization allows an individual to carry on with the intended activity for the intended time. The physiological changes are both acute (immediate to hours) and delayed (hours to days or more). Acclimatization to high altitude involves a complex series of physiological changes, including changes in ventilation, changes in pulmonary artery pressure, changes in cardiac output, changes in red cell number, changes in the number of capillaries in muscle and altered control of fluid balance

1.1   High Altitude Ascent: A Socio-economic Problem

Apart from permanent residence high altitudes is also visited by a large number of individuals for recreational purposes like skiing, mountaineering; amplifying sporting prowess through high altitude training; religious pilgrimages and also to safeguard the national territories on military front. Altitudes have always been foreseen as one of the most beautiful creations of nature and always admired. But the darker side also exists, especially when, people from sea level (or low altitudes) ascent to an altitude beyond 2500 m at a rapid rate. In such conditions high altitude poses its own set of risks and challenges to the human physique and psyche, culminating in several ailments and in worst scenarios, death. The major cause for these ill effects that has been revealed in many scientific studies is reduction in the partial pressure of air (hypobaric hypoxia) causing altered cardiopulmonary responses associated pathophysiology thereof.

Although, no distinct geological boundary exists between high altitude and low altitude, but from the scientific evidences on altitude related sickness, high altitude is considered as 1500 m above mean sea level (MSL). Further, it has been classified in three strata high altitude, 1500-3500 m, very high altitude 3500-5500 m and extreme altitude > 5500 m.[1] The highest altitude noted on the lithosphere is 8,848 meters (Mount Everest) and has been attraction for mountaineers. Figure 1.1 illustrates major Indian high attitude location with relative changes in the atmospheric pressure. (Figure 1.1). Several other mountains in the Himalayas, Swiss Alps and Andes have altitude reaching 6,096 meters (20,000 ft), and numerous tourist attractions in the altitude range of 3000 – 5000 m. As one moves to a higher altitude, the rate air becomes sparse due to lower atmospheric pressure and thereby causing decreased partial pressure of oxygen. The rate of decrease in atmospheric pressure is exponential (Peacock et al., 1998).

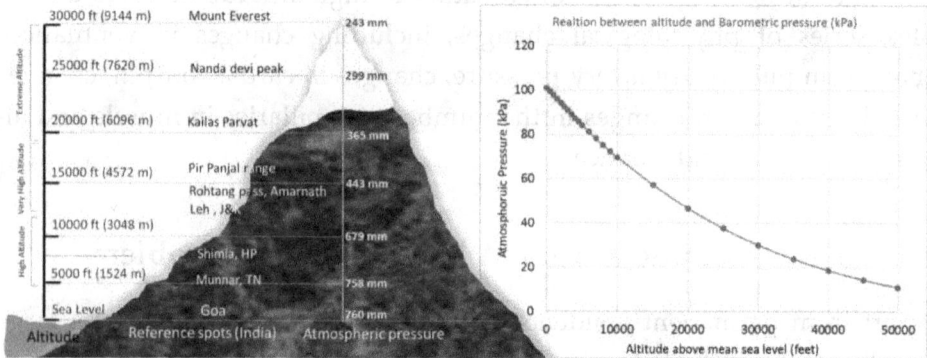

Figure 1.1: High altitude and changes in relative atmospheric pressure, Altitude above 5000 feet is considered high altitude, 11500 ft – 18000 ft as very high altitude and 18000- beyond is considered as extreme altitude (some reference tourist locations are mentioned from Indian terrain). The barometric pressure drops exponentially with increase in altitude (right panel). (Redrawn in Indian context after Radak et al., 2004).

The reduction in partial pressure of oxygen results in decreased alveolar pO2 and therefore reduced concentration of oxygen at cellular level. When alveolar partial pressure of oxygen (PAO$_2$) is normal, there is rapid diffusion of oxygen molecules through the alveolar capillary membrane into the red blood cells (RBCs) and then into combination with hemoglobin. At rest, time course for the transit of a RBC through a pulmonary capillary is of the order of 0.75 s. At sea level, breathing air within 0.25 s the oxygen tension in the blood within the capillary approaches that found within the alveoli.[2] However, at altitude PAO_2 is reduced so the rate of rise of oxygen tension within capillary blood is slower than at sea level (Figure 2.4). At rest, the capillary transit time is still sufficient to allow the oxygen tension to approach that within the alveoli, but when the transit time is reduced by exercise there will be a marked worsening of any hypobaric hypoxia.

1.2   Scientific Achievements and Clinical Landmarks

Over the past five decades, hypobaric hypoxia has been unraveled to a large extent in terms of pathophysiology, prevention and treatment. First by clinical observations then physiological observations leading to cellular, biochemical, molecular genetics and proteomics based investigations and insights. Physiological aspects such as hyperventilatory response, pulmonary vasoconstriction and cardiac hypertrophy in hypobaric hypoxia are now clearly linked with several downstream molecular cascades such as inflammatory axis, nitric-oxide dependent vasoconstriction, perturbation of cell cycle, apoptotic response and most importantly radical generation and oxidative stress. Significant amount of research has supported these evidence and therefore many research groups are also seeking newer therapeutic and prophylactic strategies based on targeting aforesaid molecular steps.

1.3   Ongoing Research and Current Challenges

Current research on hypobaric hypoxia across several research laboratories across the globe is focused on understanding the underlying molecular mechanisms and biomarker discovery aimed at early diagnosis of pathological conditions. However, a research of more than a decade have provided some of the key lead molecule for as potent biomarkers. The understanding of molecular cascades during hypobaric hypoxia have also been delineated to great extent. The major challenge is however, the variability in samples and pathophysiological response of individuals based on the differences in their genetic makeup, ethnicity and other epigenetic factors. Therefore a parallel set of studies evaluating the genomics of the high altitude response is also being carried out to associate the factors such as single nucleotide polymorphism (SNPs), copy number variation (CNVs) and restriction fragment length polymorphism to correlate with the newer discoveries pertaining to biomarker discovery. Despite of these achievement we are still far from the validated biomarker which could aid early diagnosis of acute mountain sickness.

2

Understanding High Altitude Sickness: From Pathophysiology to Underlying Cellular Changes

At low atmospheric pressure, partial pressure of oxygen (pO2) also decreases, which adversely affects human physiology (Rick, 1995) leading to high altitude illness. Rate of ascent determines the severity of illness. The symptoms usually arise within 48 h of arriving at high altitude. The common symptoms include headache, breathlessness, fatigue, nausea and vomiting, inability to sleep and swelling of face, hands and feet (Hultgren, 1996). Although it is difficult to keep the global record of high altitude sickness, yet the emerging networking and informatics tools have allowed the collection to be integrated. One such integration of data on high altitude illness was performed by Hackett and coworkers in 2004 that reported global sampling of high altitude sickness [3]

Hypoxia also causes a sequence of physiologic changes that help the body to adapt or acclimatize to the conditions. Successful acclimatization allows an individual to carry on with the intended activity for the intended time. The physiological changes are both acute (immediate to hours) and delayed (hours to days or more). Acclimatization to high altitude involves a complex series of physiological changes, including changes in ventilation, changes in pulmonary artery pressure, changes in cardiac output, changes in red cell number, changes in the number of capillaries in muscle and altered control of fluid levels.

The fine balance between the adaptability at high altitude and ill effects of hypoxia is a prime criteria of body's physiological state. Some individuals by virtue of rapid and successful adaptability cope up with hypoxia, while other which have poor adaptability, primarily due to genetic predisposition remain physiologically compromised and suffer from high altitude sickness.

In this chapter we will focus on basic understanding of high altitude sickness from the pathophysiology to underlying molecular events. Hypoxia is known to affect basic circuitry of cellular networks which included the effect on cell cycle pathways (described as separate subhead). Moreover the generation of reactive oxygen species during hypoxia is another major event that dictates the changes in pathophysiology. Also, the chapter concludes with known proteins directly involved hypoxia signalling.

2.1   Pathophysiology

Rapid ascent to high altitude is associated with physiological changes such as breathlessness, drowsiness, poor appetite (often associated with nausea), poor sleep, lassitude, insomnia, fatigue and irritability to the severe life-threatening conditions such as high-altitude pulmonary oedema (HAPE) and high-altitude cerebral oedema (HACE). The mechanisms of AMS are unknown, but rapid ascent and duration of exposure are critical. It requires an exposure of few hours to develop AMS, but it has been reported at altitudes as low as 2500 m (8000 ft) and with exposures as short as 12 h. The development of ultra-long-haul flights may increase the incidence of AMS as a flight-related condition. Once the symptoms of mountain sickness develop, the subject should go no higher, but should rest at the altitude achieved for at least 24 h. Provided that the symptoms resolve completely, the subject can then recommence climbing at a slow pace [4]. HAPE is associated with tachycardia, tachypnea and crackles in the lung bases with a dry cough. HACE is severe form of AMS with progression to ataxia, hallucinations, coma and eventually death. If symptoms suggestive of HAPE or HACE are encountered, the individual should be given oxygen and immediately descend. HAPE was first described by Ravenhill in 1913.[5] HAPE develops within 2–4 days of arrival at high altitude and is characterized by symptoms such as dyspnea at rest, decreased exercise tolerance and chest tightness. Some other signs associated with HAPE are rales or wheezing in at least one lung fluid, central cyanosis, resting tachycardia and tachypnea (Hackett et al., 1992).[6] Fever and hemoptysis may also occur. Findings on chest radiography can be variable, but usually include patchy alveolar infiltrates, which may become diffuse as the disease progresses[7, 8]. Although the exact mechanism of HAPE is not well understood, but some suggested mechanism include, an exaggerated hypoxic pulmonary vaso-constriction with an abnormal increase in pulmonary artery[9-11]. This further leads to irregular distribution of vasoconstriction with regional over perfusion [12] and increased capillary pressure [13] finally causing trans-microvascular fluid leakage[14, 15].

HACE is a potentially fatal neurological syndrome that develops over hours to days in persons with AMS or HAPE and is considered the end stage of AMS. HACE can occur 3 to 5 days after arrival to elevations as low as 2750m (9022 ft) but is most commonly seen in remote environments well above this altitude where the onset of symptoms may be much more abrupt over a period of hours. The clinical diagnosis of HACE is based on its cardinal features such as change in consciousness and ataxia [16]. Mental status changes may include irrational behaviour that rapidly progress to lethargy, obtundation and coma. Other physical signs of HACE useful in clinical diagnosis are papilledema, retinal hemorrhages, cranial nerve palsies, abnormal reflexes, and focal neurologic deficits. The exaggerated form of these clinical conditions leads to brain herniation which causes death in HACE patients[9, 17, 18]. The intracranial pressure, cerebrovascular and MRI studies have given a greater understanding of gross changes with hypobaric hypoxia but much is unknown about the mechanisms of these changes at the vascular and cellular levels.

Onset and progression of high altitude sickness may be categorized into three steps, (a) hypoxia stimulus, (b) sensing, and (c) molecular changes. Hypoxia is the primary stimulus since the initiation of pathogenesis of acute mountain sickness, although symptoms become visible 6-7 hours after the exposure, but worsen with increasing altitude [19] and relieved by normalizing the inspired PO_2[20]. These stimuli are sensed by cellular oxygen sensing system and thereby evoking compensatory response. Two major compensatory events are evoked, increased pressure (mechanical) and increased permeability (molecular). Increased permeability is regulated by potent vasodilators such as nitric oxide (NO) while pressure is increased due to hyperventilatory response. These two changes adversely affect the cardiopulmonary and cerebral systems by increased capillary pressure resulting in accumulation of fluids in brain and lung causing high altitude cerebral edema (HACE) and high altitude pulmonary edema

(HAPE) respectively (Figure 2.1). Another feature that worsens the condition is generation of radicals thereby causing oxidative stress, especially reaction between superoxide and nitric oxide producing peroxynitrite – a potent reactive molecule that causes localized histological damage.

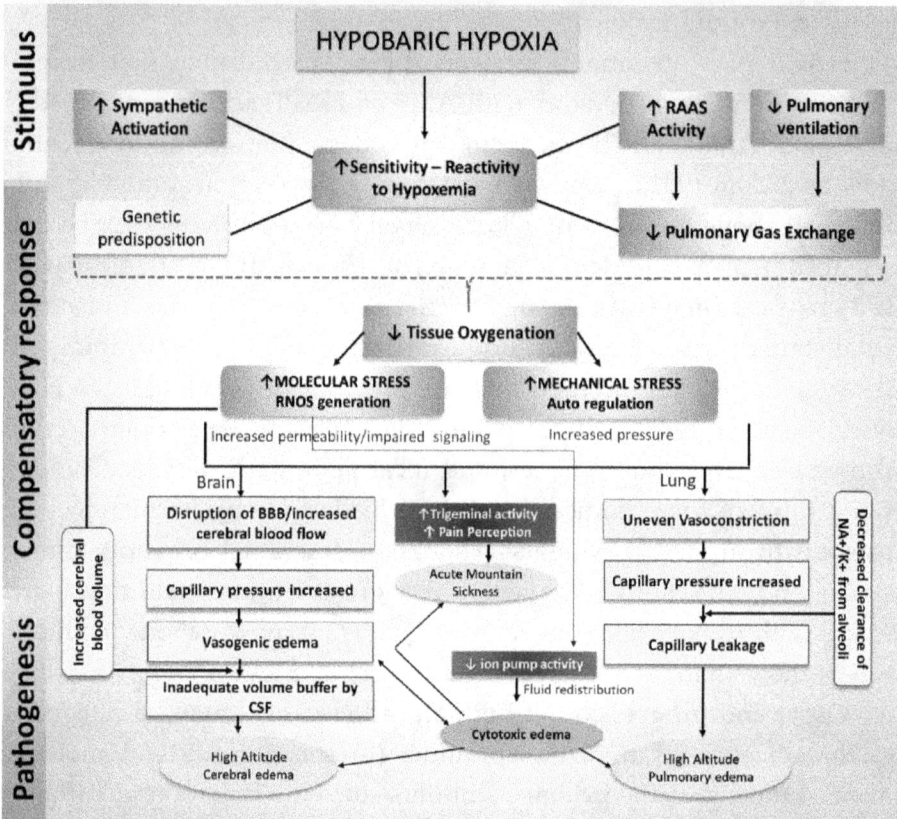

Figure 2.1: Illustration of hypobaric hypoxia induced pathophysiological changes. Initially low oxygen stimulus (hypoxia) is sensed and body evokes a compensatory response, which culminated in altered physiology and generation of RNOS, finally causing HAPE, HACE and AMS.

2.2   Hypoxia Induced Molecular Signaling

More than 90% of the total cellular oxygen uptake is recoursed to the mitochondria for oxidative phosphorylation and therefore mitochondria has been referred as an efficacious and robust oxygen sensor that can control and coordinate a variety of hypoxia responses including the HIF activity. Many studies report PHDs (Prolyl hydroxylase's) as plausible oxygen sensors, though apparently a little ambiguous. Accomplishment of this function requires PHDs to have Km in the hypoxic region. Recombinant prolyl hydroxylase's have a Km of ambient air in vitro, implying an abatement in the Prolyl hydroxylase activity as oxygen levels decline during the hypoxic conditions. Hence, if PHD's were oxygen sensors one would find a continuous increase in HIF1α agglomeration as the oxygen level falls from 21% to 0.1%, however HIF1α protein accumulation begins at ~5% oxygen and invariably increases as the oxygen levels reach up to near anoxia.[21-23]

Roles of mitochondria as oxygen sensors as well as HIF stabilizers was demonstrated by experiments on respiration-incompetent rho 0 (rho (0)) cells. Culturing cells in relatively low levels of Ethidium Bromide (EtBr) has been a procedure for generating cells that are exiguous in mitochondrial DNA and as a consequence these cells lack a functional Electron Transport Chain (ETC). Further experiments using fibroblast cells from patients with Leigh's Syndrome (Complex IV deficient) as well as cell deficient in cytochrome b/c along with depleted Rieske Iron Sulphur Protein (RISP) showed that complex III is perhaps the oxygen sensor and the results also indicate that complex III is likely involved in stabilization of HIF1α in a ROS dependent manner.[24, 25]

These experiments also showed that ROS in hypoxia is generated mainly by complex III. Although complex I and II also generate superoxide ions into the mitochondrial matrix, it is complex III which releases superoxide into the mitochondrial intermembrane space and subsequently into the cytosol and therefore contributes as the main source of ROS production in hypoxia.[23]

Literature has a lot of ambiguity about data for ROS production when measured by using conventional probes. Some laboratories showed a decrease in the ROS production while some suggested an increase during cellular hypoxia. However, with the use of advanced sensitive ROS scanning systems based on oxidation of sensitive proteins coupled to fluorescence energy transfer like HSP FRET and roGFP, a clear picture indicating an increase in the ROS levels during hypoxia has been observed in a majority of cell systems. Biologically, ROS is derived from either superoxide or hydrogen peroxide with varied cellular sources ranging from mitochondria, ER to peroxisomes and plasma membrane.

Ubiquinone (Q) cycle of complex III is the cardinal primary element for ROS generation during hypoxia and also plays an integral role in HIF 1α stabilization. The Q cycle is set in motion when complex I and II transfer electrons to reduce the lipid moiety ubiquinone to ubiquinol which subsequently enters the Q cycle. The first step in Q cycle is the transfer of electrons to the Rieske Fe-S protein which oxidises Ubiquinol (QH2) to Ubi semiquinone (QHo) at the Qo site of complex III. This electron is transferred to cytochrome c1, which in turn reduces cytochrome c. Further, complex IV oxidises cytochrome c followed by transfer of electrons to molecular oxygen and ultimately reduction to water. This pathway accounts for one electron that reduced Ubiquinone to Ubiquinol and at this point the Q cycle is only half complete because the other electron is still maintained by the highly reactive intermediate Ubi semiquinone.

Ubi semiquinone quickly reduces the bL reaction centre of cytochrome b at the Qo site of complex III. Electron is then passed from the bL reaction centre to the bH reaction centre of cytochrome b. The electron from the bH reaction centre reduces either ubiquinone or semi ubiquinone at the Qi site of complex III and when the electron is passed to Rieske Fe-S protein and cytochrome c1, the Q cycle is effectuated. Ubi semiquinone is a highly reactive intermediate that is procreated at the Qo site. As a repercussion of electron transfer through the Q cycle, ubi semiquinone can generate superoxide at the Qo site and the same has been confirmed by many pharmacological interventions which indicate that the Qo site is mainly responsible for generation of ROS during hypoxia.[26-28] HIF is an important historical transcription factor which associates with specific nuclear factors under hypoxia to transactivate a passel of genes to trigger adaptive as well as beyond adaptive responses in low oxygen tensions. This PER-ARNT-SIM family of transcription factor plays a central role in hypoxia response, yet there are many reports that suggest its role to be less important and rather arguable in hypoxia biology.

As per canonical HIF pathway, in well oxygenated conditions (normoxia), PHD dependent hydroxylation of two proline residues (P-402 and P-564) in the oxygen dependent degradation domain (ODD) of HIF1α, allows its specific recognition by pVHL E3 Ligase complex leading to its degradation by 26S proteasomal complex. However, as oxygen is one of the vital cofactors required for PHD to function, therefore, during low oxygen concentrations, HIF is not hydroxylated and hence stabilized.[29] When subjected to hypoxia, HIF activates the transcription of over 40 genes, including erythropoietin, glucose transporters, glycolytic enzymes, vascular endothelial growth factor, HILPDA, and other genes whose protein products augment oxygen delivery or facilitate as well as assist in the metabolic adaptation to hypoxia.[30] HIF has also been suggested to personate vital roles in embryonic vascularization, tumour angiogenesis and pathophysiology of ischemic disease.[31-33] But the above experimental indications and findings do not rationalize some of the important findings which have been reported every year regarding "HIF not being the sole master regulator transcription factor in hypoxia, also HIF being a very generalised transcription factor which is activated in diverse conditions via different mechanisms and therefore not restricted to hypoxia". Some key findings have been summarised below.[34] Mature monocytes normalize towards sites of inflammation and infection where they differentiate into inflammatory macrophages or into dendritic cells. Hypoxic environment has been a hallmark of inflammatory regions as well as malignant tumours. Neither HIF1α/2α/3α was found by Elbarghati *et al.* in primary monocytes after hypoxia incubation for 24hrs.[35] Authors hypothesized that HIFα subunits are not expressed because monocytes usually reside in peripheral blood which usually contains very high oxygen levels. They also reported that primary human macrophages but not monocytes rapidly upregulated HIF1α/2α proteins upon exposure to hypoxia along with nuclear translocation.[36]

Further it has been reported that NFκB, a transcription factor regulated by hypoxia is involved in the adaptive response of primary monocytes to hypoxia. Even TLR stimulation has not been found to affect HIF1α localisation in monocytes. HIF1α accumulates in quiescent human monocytes under hypoxia, but solely in the cytoplasm and therefore it cannot function as a transcription factor. Reports suggest that HIF1α dependent gene regulation can be a feature of evolutionarily young cells of the adaptive immune system, but not of the old cells of innate immune system such as monocytes.[36] During differentiation of human monocytes to macrophages, more potent and robust HIF system is activated due to nuclear translocation. This may be regarded as an adaptation for a nomadic life style of macrophages which constantly work in low oxygen areas. Therefore, these results show that HIF mediated gene regulation is not a "by rule" in hypoxia physiology.

There are reports which suggest that macrophages require stable HIF1α levels for regular ATP maintenance and HIF1α null cells in normoxia have ~80% low ATP levels. Therefore, it can be inferred that HIF1α stabilization is just not a hypoxic phenomenon. There have been meaningful affirmations for HIF induction by non-hypoxic stimuli, specifically in cases of oncogenic mutation (ras, src, PTEN), growth factor stimulations i.e. insulin, insulin like growth factor-I and EGF[37,38] and NO[39]. Other stimuli that bring about normoxic HIF stabilization in macrophages include low density lipoproteins and macrophage derived peptide PR39. It is therefore likely that a complex growth factor rich environment can cause HIF induction/stabilization. Even in the tissue culture models of macrophage differentiation, it has been shown that HIF1α accumulates in phorbol-12-myristate 13 acetate (PMA) differentiated THP1 and U937 cells and this is coincident with a marked curtailment in the intracellular iron pool.[40]

Some groups have found that adenosine and A2a receptor via protein kinase C and PI3K dependent pathways cause normoxic induction of HIF1α in macrophages.[41] A lot of disparity has been seen in non- hypoxic HIF1α induction as compared with the hypoxic conditions, as in normoxia the stabilization of HIF1α (via PHD mediated pathway) does not seem to be for its functionality but the predominant mechanism in normoxia being an increase in HIF1α protein translation which is in turn mediated centrally by PI3K pathway. There is also evidence of increase in HIF1α mRNA levels. Adenosine treatment has been found to induce HIF1α binding activity, nuclear assemblage and transactivation capacity by activation of A2A receptors in J774A.1 mouse macrophages under normoxia.[41] A similar finding was observed in adenosine treated mouse peritoneal macrophages.

Normoxic HIF1α activation through ROS generation via angiotensin II stimulation has also been reported in vascular smooth muscle cells. The prime source of ROS here has been the complex III of mitochondria. Previous reports indicate that neutralising ROS with antioxidants allows HIF1α protein to remain hydroxylated under hypoxic condition and therefore invigorates it for degradation. Also, at the same time increasing ROS levels under normoxia by over expressing glucose oxidase stopped normoxic HIF1α protein hydroxylation and therefore prevents its degradation. Loss of Jun D, a member of AP-1 family of transcription factors increases the oxidative stress in cells and also results in normoxic activation of HIF1α and VEGF.[42]

Atkuri *et al.* showed that culturing primary T lymphocytes at atmospheric oxygen (which we usually do) shifts and distorts the intracellular redox state. Freshly taken out PBMC's have been compared with T cells cultured for 3 days at atmospheric oxygen as well as physiological oxygen (5%) without exogenous stimuli. GSH (iGSH) vs. oxidized GSH (iGSH) was measured by tandem MS and a loss of GSH at both atmospheric and physiological oxygen in T cells was observed. However, the maximum loss was found in T cells grown in atmospheric oxygen. Significantly high levels of iGSSG were observed in primary T cells cultured at atmospheric oxygen in comparison to those cultured at physiological oxygen (1.5-2.0 folds). Therefore, GSH/GSSG ratio was significantly high for cells cultured at physiological oxygen and substantially reduced in case cells grown at atmospheric oxygen. Thus, implications of ROS generation and oxidative stress in cells cultured at atmospheric oxygen are prominent. Redox state of freshly isolated cells and those grown at physiological oxygen were much closer. So, from these experiments we speculate that there are relatively high levels of ROS when primary cells are grown at 21% and therefore as described above that ROS levels increase HIF activation, it is very much possible that cells grown at normoxia may have high HIF activation as well as induction and therefore at times can be very misleading.[43]

In another important study, Frede *et al.* reported that in monocytes and macrophages, bacterial LPS induces HIF mRNA and protein accumulation in both primary (human) cells as well as cell lines like THP-1 under normoxic conditions. LPS increases HIF1α via NFκB involving MAPK P44/42 pathway. NFκB site has been implicated in the promoter of HIF1α gene and is therefore an important mechanism in normoxic HIF stabilization. This also further implicates that bacterial infections can lead to HIF stabilization.[44]

Another very important event in HIF biology reported by Benizri *et al.* (2008) is HIF de sensitization where HIF1α/2α levels decay due to unforeseen and gradual PHD over-activation in chronic hypoxia regardless of low global oxygen. Chronic hypoxia therefore is neither able to amass HIF1α nor HIF2α in many of the cell systems seen so far by re-establishing PHD-VHL proteasome degradation pathway. Chronic hypoxia over activates three PHD's.[45]

2.3   Hypoxia and Cell Cycle Regulation

For unicellular organisms, the decision to enter the cell cycle can be essentially viewed as a metabolically active process. A cell must assess its nutritional and metabolic status to ensure that it can synthesize sufficient biomass to produce a new daughter cell. The cell must then direct the appropriate metabolic outputs to ensure completion of the division process.

Cell division is one of the important fundamental biological processes regulated by oxygen availability. For most cell types, hypoxia causes a decrease in the rate of cell division/ cell proliferation since an increase in cell number would further lead to an increase the oxygen consumption, thus, resulting in even more severe hypoxia. On the other hand, certain specialized cell types are likely to undertake mitotic process under hypoxic conditions e.g. during angiogenesis which requires proliferation of vascular endothelial cells.[32] Primary mouse cells i.e. embryonic fibroblasts were found to have decreased Brdu incorporation with respect to 20% O_2 after 24 h of hypoxia (0.5% O_2).[46] This effect was observed in the wild type and p53-/- cells. However, Brdu incorporation was not observed to be inhibited when HIF1α deficient fibroblasts were cultured under hypoxic conditions. At the same time over-expression of HIF1α was found to increase p21 and block Brdu incorporation in human HCT116 cells cultured under non-hypoxic conditions.[47]

Transcription factor c-myc interacts with MIZ1 bound to the initiator element of CDKN1A promoter to repress transcription of CDKN1A gene (which encodes for p21)[48] and thus, increase cell proliferation[49]. The binding of c-Myc has been reported in cells cultured under non-hypoxic conditions while HIF1α has been found to replace c-Myc for binding in cells exposed to hypoxic state. This decreased c-Myc binding causes a derepression of CDKN1 transcription, which in turn leads to an increase in the p21 levels. Additionally, the effect of HIF1α has been observed to be independent of HRE and HIF1β in such conditions. Forced over expression of HIF1α is sufficient to arrest the cell cycle. Prior to the onset of DNA replication, formation of pre- replicative complex occurs during the G1 phase and loading of MCM (MCM 2-7) onto the origin is referred to as replication licensing.[50] MCM helicases form an important part of the pre-replication complex. HIF1α and MCM function together in a mutually antagonistic manner. MCM causes an inhibition of the HIF activity via oxygen dependent hydroxylation by giving more stability to the HIF1α-Vhl- Elongin C complex.[51] However, the capacity of HIF1α to slow down/inhibit cell cycle progression under severe hypoxia can outweigh the ability of MCM to promote cell cycle progression since hydroxylation is inhibited under the case of severe hypoxia wherein oxygen as a substrate is very limited. Individual MCM act as HIF inhibitors rather than the full complex and therefore, their role as inhibitors are much more prominent than helicases.[52]

In cardiac fibroblasts, P38 MAPK regulates G1-S transition during hypoxia. These cells are important for myocardial repair subsequent to an injury as they are a rich source of extracellular matrix proteins, matrix metalloproteases and several growth factors. Quiescent cardiac fibroblasts undergo transformations in the phenotype after myocardial injury which either leads to their exit or entry into the cell cycle. These fibroblasts may also turn into activated myofibroblasts. Their entry/exit from the cell cycle can affect the outcome of various diseases e.g. Myocardial Infarction, since these cells play a major role in myocardial remodelling. Hypoxia is a major constituent of several disease states of the myocardium. G1-S check point is very critical and is driven by cyclin dependent kinase complexes including Cyclin D (CDK4/6) and Cyclin E (CDK2) that phosphorylate Rb protein facilitating S phase entry. Inhibition of CDK activity by cyclin dependent kinase inhibitors such as p21 and p27 promotes Rb hypophosphorylation and thus, the cell cycle gets arrested.[53,54] Reduced levels of cyclin D/A and induction of p27 has been experimentally validated in hypoxic conditions and has been found to result in hypophosphorylation of Rb under hypoxia. Levels of SKP2, which targets p27 for degradation, have been observed to be very low during hypoxia. Furthermore, they have also been found to show an inverse relationship with p27.

Molecular mechanisms discussed in the preceding sections show how cells adapt to a low oxygen environment. However, literature suggests that such low oxygen conditions can induce apoptosis, when oxygen levels decrease to or below 0.5%. When oxygen levels are between 0.5% – 3%, the cells generally do not undergo apoptosis, instead hypoxia activates a variety of cellular adaptive events which lead to cell survival. Therefore, it can be inferred that low oxygen concentration triggers both cell death and survival pathways, depending on the percentage and time of exposure. Subjection to severe and prolonged hypoxia may initiate apoptosis or necrosis while mild hypoxia is protective in nature. In fact mild hypoxia interferes with several components of the apoptotic pathway at the transcriptional as well as at the post translational level. Hypoxia driven apoptosis is by far a result of the dominance of apoptotic factors over adaptive factors and some upstream signalling molecules have been found to regulate the fate of cell in hypoxia. Some molecules have been found to be anti-apoptotic in certain cell systems and apoptotic in the others whereas some get too exhausted in the chronic conditions to provide resistance leading to an apoptotic phenotype. Henceforth, it can be concluded that the apoptotic phenotype is actually a result of complex cellular signalling. One of the important organelle associated with apoptotic signalling is "mitochondria". Interestingly, A549 cells devoid of mitochondrial DNA ($\rho 0$ cells) and also lacking a functional Electron Transport Chain (ETC) are resistant to anoxia induced apoptosis.[55] Loss of ATP is also a very important factor for hypoxia induced cell death. Once the ATP levels deplete profoundly, progressive cell death follows and to a great extent it is the adaptive hypoxic responses that play a major role in maintaining the ATP for cell survival. However, after a certain time of exposure or limit of oxygen, these adaptive mechanisms fails to counteract the low oxygen mediated energy loss and therefore, the cells are unable to preserve the minimum threshold of energy needed for cell survival.

2.4   ROS Generation during Hypoxia

Hypobaric hypoxia induces oxidative stress with an increased production of reactive oxygen species (ROS) and contributes to mechanisms of vascular dysfunction. Oxidative stress is mainly caused by an imbalance between the activity of endogenous pro-oxidative enzymes (such as NADPH oxidase, xanthine oxidase, or the mitochondrial respiratory chain) and anti-oxidative enzymes (such as superoxide dismutase, glutathione peroxidase, heme oxygenase, thioredoxin peroxidase/peroxiredoxin, catalase, and paraoxonase) [56]. Hypobaric hypoxia works in favour of the former. This allows the accumulation of reactive oxygen species (ROS) in the physiological system. Major enzymes involved in ROS generation in vasculature are NADPH oxidase, xanthine oxidase, a dysfunctional eNOS (in which oxygen reduction is uncoupled from NO synthesis), and enzymes of the mitochondrial respiratory chain.[57] Reactive species and free radicals like peroxides, superoxides are oxygen centred molecules which are unstable (e.g., having unpaired electron) and promote oxidation reactions with other molecules, such as proteins, lipids, and DNA, in order to become stabilized.[58,59] Free radicals and ROS have various regulatory roles in cells and are essential to our wellbeing. For example, ROS are produced by immune cells (neutrophils and macrophages) in the process of respiratory burst protect cells by eliminating antigens.[60] ROS also serve as stimulating signals for several genes which encode transcription factors, differentiation, and development as well as stimulating cell-cell adhesion, cell signaling, involvement in vasoregulation and fibroblast proliferation, and increased expression of antioxidant enzymes.[61] Details of molecules majorly involved in ROS generation are mentioned below:

(a) NADPH Oxidase

NADPH oxidases (Nox) are multi-component enzymes exist in membranes endothelial cells, smooth muscle cells, and fibroblasts and several other types of cells. Studies have shown that NADPH is involved in angiotensin II-induced hypertension [62,63], diabetes mellitus [64], and hypercholesterolemia [65], and atherosclerosis [66]. Nox1-deficient mice show smaller blood pressure increases to angiotensin II [62]. whereas mice overexpressing Nox1 in smooth muscle showed greater blood pressure responses to angiotensin II and increased $O_2 \cdot^\bullet$ production [67].

(b) Respiratory Chain of the Mitochondria

Mitochondria consume about 1% oxygen and the "leakage" of activated oxygen from mitochondria during oxidative respiration is important sources of $O_2 \cdot^\bullet$ in the cardiovascular system[56]. Mitochondrial $O_2\cdot^\bullet$ production is associated with complex I and III of the respiratory chain. Complex I (iron-sulphur clusters) releases the reactive oxygen species- superoxide anion only towards the mitochondrial matrix, whereas complex III (ubiquinol oxidation site) releases superoxide into both matrix and outside the inner membrane[68]. Dysregulated free radical generation leads to the development of cardiovascular dysfunctions and early atherosclerotic lesions[69,70]. Mitochondrial dysfunction, resulting from SOD2 deficiency, increases mitochondrial DNA (mtDNA) damage and accelerates atherosclerosis in apoE -/- mice[71].

(c) Uncoupled NOS/eNOS

Nitric oxide synthase normally involved in multifunctional NO. However, NOS/eNOS itself act as a source of superoxide as electron transfer in NOS enzymes is tightly controlled to NO synthesis. Imbalance between electron transfer and NO generation results in NOS uncoupling turning the functional NOS into a dysfunctional $O_2^{-\cdot}$ generating enzyme[72]. Several studies provide the evidence for eNOS uncoupling like in high altitude induced pulmonary arterial hypertension[73], peroxynitrite-treated rat aorta in endothelial cells treated with low-density lipoprotein[74], and in isolated blood vessels of spontaneously hypertensive rats[75], stroke-prone spontaneously hypertensive rats[76] and angiotensin II-induced hypertension[77]. eNOS uncoupling has also been seen in patients with endothelial dysfunction due to hypercholesterolemia[78] diabetes mellitus[79] and essential hypertension[80].

There are studies which showed that high altitude (4000m) exposure resulted in decreased activity and protein content of mitochondrial SOD in skeletal muscle of rats[58], but 5500m simulated altitude increased the level immunoreactive MnSOD in the serum and decreased it in liver and lung of the animals. The activity of glutathione peroxidase (GPx) also decreased in liver suggesting that liver might especially sensitive to high altitude induced oxidative stress.[81] High altitude exposure decreases the level of reduced glutathione (GS) and increase oxidized glutathione concentration.[82,83] Simulated high altitude at 25000m for 2 day induces ROS generation in rat heart, indicated by increased lipid peroxidation, protein carbonylation and compromised antioxidant system.[84]

Antioxidant system which acts against oxidative stress includes important enzymes like superoxide dismutase (SOD), glutathione peroxidase (GPx), catalase, heme oxygenase (HO), and the thioredoxin (Trx) peroxidase perhaps also paraoxonases (PON). SOD catalyzes the dismutation of $O_2^{-\cdot}$ into oxygen and hydrogen peroxide and serve as major antioxidant. Three forms of the SOD enzyme exists in human: SOD1 (Cu-Zn-SOD) is located in the cytoplasm, SOD2 (Mn-SOD) in the mitochondria, and SOD3 (Cu-Zn-SOD) is extracellular. Catalase is another important enzyme which plays role on ROS scavenging. Similarly, GPx reduces free hydrogen peroxide to water and lipid hydroperoxides to their corresponding alcohols. Heme-oxygenase1 (HO-1) is the antioxidant enzyme which generates equimolar of carbon monoxide, bilivrdin and free ferrous iron by metabolising heme. The PON family of enzymes contribute to vascular antioxidant defense, reduces ROS generation and protect against coronary artery disease[85]. Thioredoxins (Trx) are efficient peroxynitrite (ONOO-) scavengers which is present in endothelial cells and vascular smooth muscle cells. Thioredoxin peroxidsae (peroxiredoxin) Peroxyredoxins are reduced by Trx and the reduced form of peroxiredoxins scavenges most of the H_2O_2 and ONOO-. In order to understand better, the antioxidant defence explained above could be hypothetically stratified into different strata based on their defence against radicals, this has been illustrated in Figure 2.2 below.

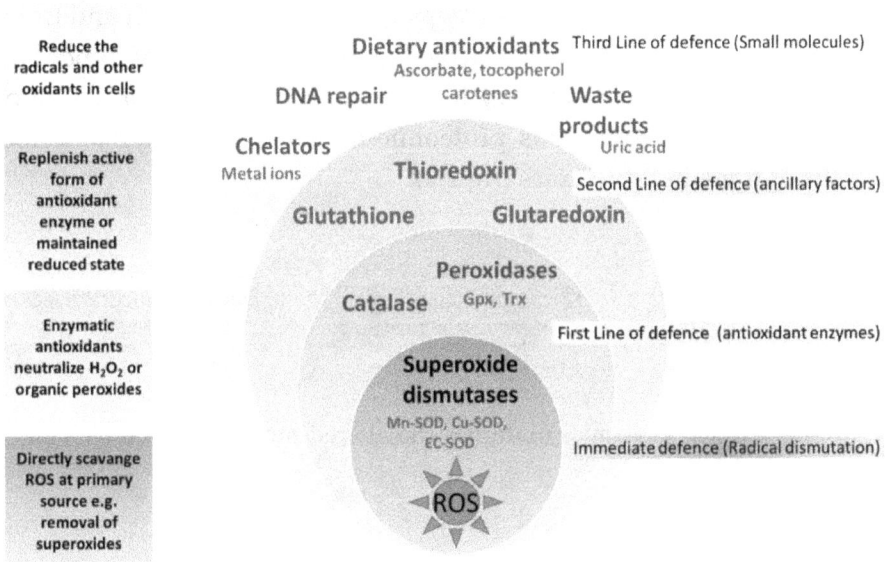

Figure 2.2: Stratification of antioxidant defence: Defense against oxidative stress: at primary level en source generation of radicals is dismutated by SOD, which further produces hydrogen peroxide and organic peroxides. These are neutralized by catalase and GSH or TRX dependent peroxidases. Glutathione, Glutaredoxin and Thioredoxin feed the maintenance of active form of enzyme and reduced state of proteins. Finally many small metabolites like uric acid, metal Chelators or even dietary antioxidants such as Ascorbate, carotenes and tocopherol scavange radicals.

2.5   Protein Dynamics Underlies the Altered Molecular Circuitry and Pathophysiology

As seen above, a plethora of molecules and intricate circuitry of molecular pathways including the biochemical pathways are affected by hypoxic stress. Changes in the expression profile, sub-cellular localization and protein interactions underlies the aforesaid molecular changes. A large number of studies on variety of cell lines, animal models and human subjects have been performed to evaluate the dynamics of proteins during hypoxic conditions. Basic information about the expression of genes can be obtained using either large scale expression profiling such as microarray or PCR arrays, however the information available from such experiments not enough perhaps due to a number of steps between transcription and translation such as si-RNA or mi-RNA mediated degradation of functional transcripts. It is therefore necessary to observe the precise information on protein dynamics using various proteomic tools. Next chapter describes basic tools of trade in proteomics (fig 2.3).

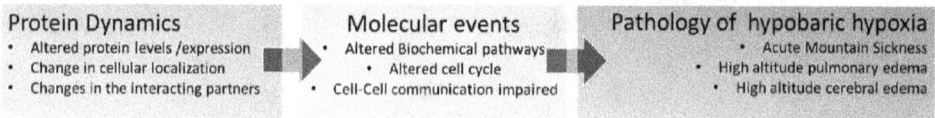

Protein Dynamics	Molecular events	Pathology of hypobaric hypoxia
• Altered protein levels /expression • Change in cellular localization • Changes in the interacting partners	• Altered Biochemical pathways • Altered cell cycle • Cell-Cell communication impaired	• Acute Mountain Sickness • High altitude pulmonary edema • High altitude cerebral edema

Figure 2.3: Protein dynamics underlies the altered molecular circuitry and pathophysiology.

3

Proteomics: Tool of trade

As discussed in the previous section, proteins form a major set of biomolecules that decide that pathophysiology of high altitude sickness dictating the importance of proteomic study. Now when the focus is switching from pathophysiology to susceptibility transcriptomics and genomics which answers the predisposition of high altitude sickness in an individual, the importance of proteins still remains, provided the spatial and temporal dynamics of proteins.

3.1   Proteome and Proteomics

Proteome was coined by Marc Wilkins, which he used for the entire complement of protein expressed by a genome, cell, tissue or organism. Proteomics is the study and characterization of complete set of proteins that are present in cell, organ, or organism at a given time[86]. Unlike genomes proteomes have both temporal and spatial variations which escalates the complexity of its study. However, this variation is important for clinical diagnosis of various pathological conditions, as a minute change in cellular or subcellular metabolism may alter its proteome[87]. Last decade has witnessed tremendous increase in the whole genome sequences. As per the recent data from genome online database (GOLD), there are 9191 eukaryotic genomes sequenced so far, while there are 38967 genomes available within bacterial domain[88]. This exponential rise is however not concurrent with proteome maps, perhaps due to lack of advent in proteome analysis technologies and also several challenges due to dynamic nature of proteomes. The dynamics of proteome is further complicated by post translational modifications that regulate the protein activity that creates a difference between proteome and functional proteome, one of the emerging field in proteomics.

Proteomics, the science that studies the global patterns of protein expression in individual cells, tissues, or body fluids, has been growing rapidly for the last few decades. However, as more studies are yielding new data with far-reaching implications, researchers are starting to look at proteomics as a new source of clues to help in the early diagnosis of disease and in prediction of clinical outcomes. Instead of tracking a single biomarker, proteomics is attempting to define global patterns of protein expression with diagnostic or prognostic value for a particular form of disease. Such data sets are obtained using large numbers of samples from patients divided in appropriate categories vs. healthy controls or patients with good prognosis, analyzed for correlation and significance, and further validated using out-of-sample clinical data.

3.2   Commonly used Techniques in Proteomics

One dimensional gel electrophoresis is based on electrophoretic mobility of proteins on an inert support such as polyacrylamide and agarose that results in separation of proteins on the basis of their molecular weight. Any shift or missing bands might represent alteration in the proteome status. Several variants of the gel electrophoresis have been developed, Native-polyacrylamide gel electrophoresis s (PAGE) involves the use of proteins in native state and therefore use of denaturing conditions such as mercaptoethanol, dithiothreitol, or sample boiling is eliminated. This technique is useful for determination of biological activity of proteins in gels.

Two dimensional electrophoresis has preceded and accompanied the birth of proteomics. Established in the early '70s by O'Farrel, 2DGE still remains the technique of choice for this kind of study although lately interest has focused on the development of gel-free techniques. The 2DE is reproducible, robust and able to best resolve a complex protein mixture according to their isoelectric point (pI) and their molecular weight (MW). The polyacrylamide gels, where the protein species are resolved, represent the "core" of the proteomic analysis. Its structure consents to physically match two different samples. Thanks to this, two different protein mixtures are compared to each other in both quantitative and qualitative points of view. Another advantage of the 2DE method is represented from the study of post-translational modifications that determined an alteration of the pI and MW inducing a positional shift in the 2D gel. This kind of modification is represented by phosphorylation, glycosylation, glutathionylation or more neglected modification such as protein cleavage. In conclusion, the 2DE for separative step is decisive for the next selection of interesting spots for the analysis. Although widely used, 2DE presents some limitations: the reduced dynamic range, for instance, allow the visualization of the under-represented proteins limiting the global approach of the proteomic method. In addition, 2D gels also rarely display hydrophobic proteins and only highly abundant proteins are currently visualized. Low abundance proteins of physiological relevance, such as regulators or signaling proteins are difficult to detect. Moreover, basic or very basic proteins are rather difficult to focus. In addition to these technical problems, 2DE is a "time-consuming" method that makes it possible to carry out a comparison of a low number of analytical and biological replicates.

In support of the various problems encountered with classical 2DE on gel-to-gel variations and time-consuming questions, DIGE has been developed which substantially reduces variability by sample labeling with different fluorescent dyes (Cy2, Cy3, and Cy5). In the same gel it is possible to resolve control and treated samples labeled independently with a fluorescent dye such as Cy3 or Cy5. Cy2 allows labeling an internal standard, a mixture containing equal amounts of each experimental sample taken into consideration. Two samples and the internal standard are mixed together and resolved in the same gel. Densitometric scanning at different wavelengths, characteristic for each dye, permit to obtain three images from only one gel, two from samples and one from internal standard. This procedure allows a very accurate and fast computer analysis reducing errors due to the distortion of the experimental gels. The internal standard represents the average of the analyzed samples reporting every protein species. Its use allows an accurate statistical spot quantification as well as an increase in matching gel reliability to distinguish the experimental from biological variations in the samples. The classical or DIGE gel production needs an image analysis step by dedicated software such as Image Master 2D Platinum (GE Healthcare, Uppsala, Sweden) for classical gels and DeCyder (DeCyder Differential Analysis software, GE Healthcare) with regard to the DIGE gels. The usefulness of DIGE is amplified multifold by the use of mass spectrometry.

Mass spectrometry (MS) is based on the identification of a molecule on the basis of small molecular fragments created by high energy laser and detected on the basis of their different mass to charge (m/z) ratios. MS was classically a tool for chemists for the identification of relatively smaller molecules however the usefulness of mass spectrometry was focused in early 90s when Tanaka *et al.*, demonstrated the identification of proteins using matrix assisted laser dissociation spectrometry (MADLI). Perhaps, this techniques should be considered as a quantum leap for the rapid growth of proteomics in the last decade[89]. In MALDI ToF procedure, the protein spot of interest resolved by 2DE, is previously subjected to hydrolytic cut by trypsin. This enzyme cuts the peptide chain at arginine and lysine levels. The obtained peptide mixture, placed in the target plate, is mixed with a matrix, composed by small aromatic rings (saturated solution of α-cyano-4-hydroxycinnamic acid). MALDI is a soft ionization technique allowing the analysis of biomolecules which tend to be fragile and fragment when ionized by more conventional ionization methods. In the first part of MALDI ToF analysis, aromatic groups of the matrix absorb the laser energy ionizing its acidic group. This process consents to transfer a proton to the peptide. The description of the sample is achieved by the vacuum in the flight tube. This process consents to obtain charged and in gaseous phase peptides that fly in the flight tube only depending on electromagnetic potential difference where every peptide will be characterized by the same kinetic energy. What distinguishes the time of flight of each peptide, that is, the time that the peptide employs to reach the detector starting from the target plate, will be its m/z ratio. Every peptide assumes a single charge ($z = +1$), hence the mass will characterize each amino acid side chain and then the time of flight. According to this, the smaller peptides will reach the detector before the bigger ones. The time of flight employed will be recorded and reported on a spectrogram, a graph showing the values of the m/z ratios on the x-axis and the intensity of each peak on the y-axis (each ion with the same m/z ratio). All the m/z values determine the peptide mass fingerprinting (PMF) of the protein, useful in comparing the experimental masses obtained from MALDI ToF, with the theoretical masses in specific databases available online on Swiss Prot (http://www.expasy.org/sprot/) and NCBInr (www.ncbi.nlm.nih.gov/protein). Mascot Search (www.matrixscience.com) is a research program, similar to Profound (http://prowl.rockefeller.edu/

profound_bin/WebProFound.exe), able to perform the comparison between experimental and theoretical masses to identify the protein. The degree of identification accuracy is estimated by score value and sequence coverage. MALDI ToF technology is extremely versatile in proteomic analysis thanks to its capacity to generate mono-charged ions and to its high sensitivity. The MALDI ToF can also be applied to the protein modification such as post-translational modification (phosphorilation, glycosylation etc) and protein interactions (protein-ligand or protein-metal ions). Later other variants of mass spectrometers based on electrospray ionization (ESI) and quadruple detectors increased the sensitivity of protein identification. In contrast to the MALDI ionization, which leads to the mono-charged ion formation, ESI ionization leads to multi charged ion formation. The HPLC and ESI-IT conjugation allows to increase the spectrometer sensitivity because it is very dependent on sample entrance flow. Nanoliters/minute flow allows to obtain high sensitivity performance.

Edman degradation, a method for proteomic sequence also emerged as an important tool in determination of proteins sequences and growth of the proteome databank pools of several organisms. However, the complex nature of technique and advent of bioinformatics tools to obtain protein sequence from genomic data downgraded the importance of protein sequencing. Currently, mass spectrometric techniques have also matured as a tool for determination for protein sequences by using MS^n.

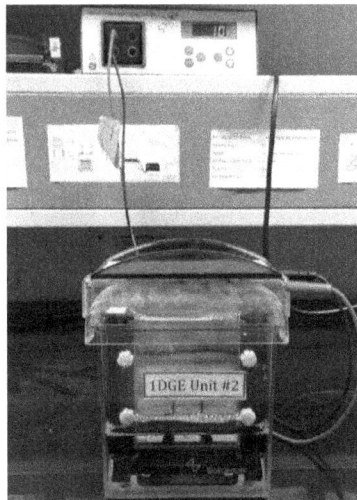

Figure 3.1: Set-up used for one dimetional gel electrophoresis.

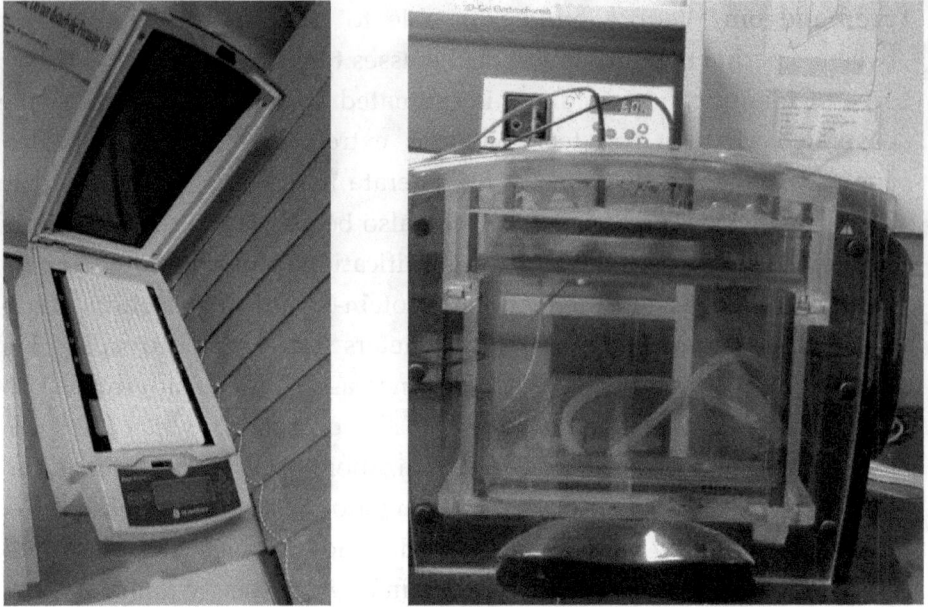

Figure 3.2: Isoelectric focusing and 2D gel electrophoresis apparatus.

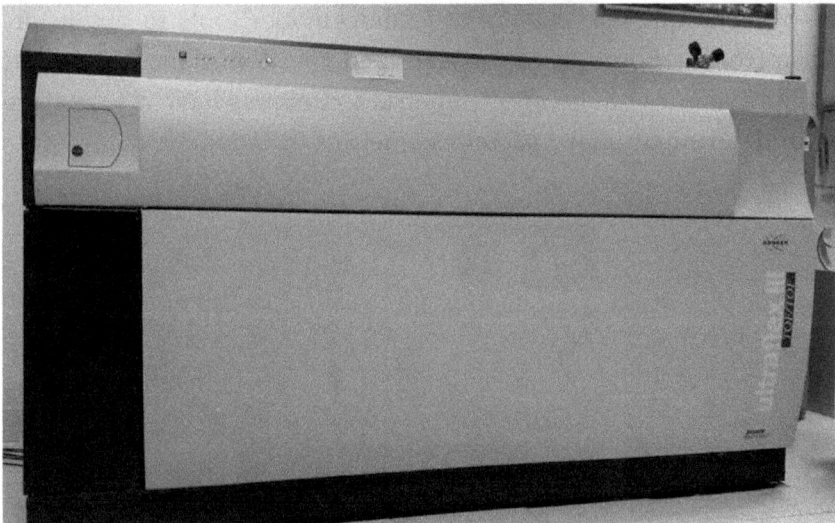

Figure 3.3: MALDI-TOF, commonly used tool for identification of proteins after 2DGE, based on the principle of ionized mass separation and spectral match with known databases.

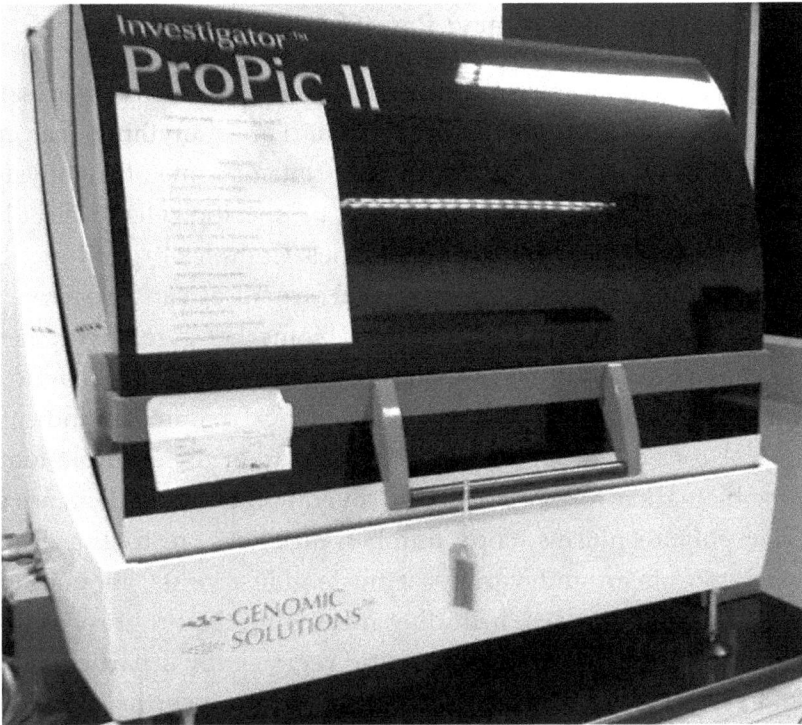

Figure 3.4: Automated spot picker used for high throughput picking of spots from 2D gels.

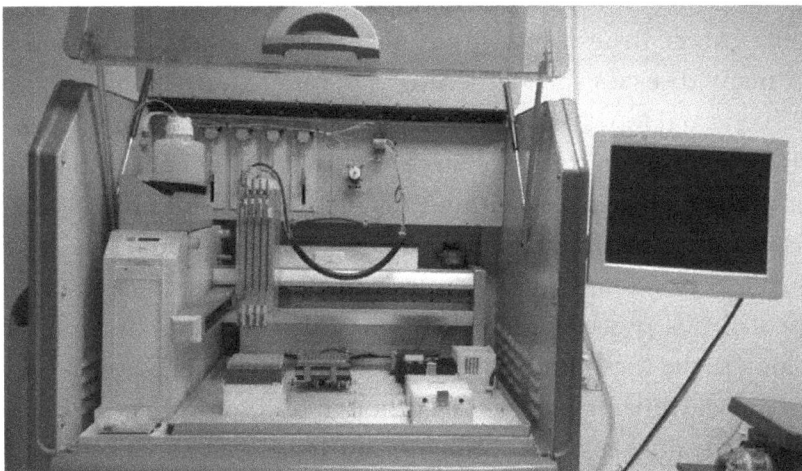

Figure 3.5: Automated gel digester used for high throughput digesting gel pieces isolated picked from 2D gels: a robotic arm based apparatus.

3.3   Biomarkers discovery: Payoff from Proteomics

Biomarker is defined as measurable indicator of the severity or presence of some disease state. More generally a biomarker is anything that can be used as an indicator of a particular disease state or some other physiological state of an organism. Biomarkers can be specific cells, molecules, or genes, gene products, enzymes, or hormones. Complex organ functions or general characteristic changes in biological structures can also serve as biomarkers (Figure 3.6). Although the term biomarker is relatively new, biomarkers have been used in pre-clinical research and clinical diagnosis for a considerable time. Even a minor physiological parameter indicating a pathological condition may be called as biomarker for example temperature is the biomarker for fever. Among several other biomarkers are single nucleotide polymorphisms, copy number variations, restriction fragment length polymorphism and variety of nucleotide repeats. Biomarkers are useful in a number of ways, including measuring the progress of disease, evaluating the most effective therapeutic regimes for a particular cancer type, and establishing long-term susceptibility to cancer or its recurrence (http://www.biomarkersconsortium.org). The parameter can be chemical, physical or biological. In molecular terms biomarker is "the subset of markers that might be discovered using genomics, proteomics technologies or imaging technologies. Biomarkers play major roles in medicinal biology. Biomarkers help in early diagnosis, disease prevention, drug target identification, drug response etc. Several biomarkers have been identified for many diseases such as serum LDL for cholesterol, blood pressure, and P53 gene and MMPs as tumor markers for cancer.[90,91]

The recent interest in biomarker discovery is enhanced by new molecular biologic techniques, without detailed insight into the mechanisms of a disease. By screening many possible biomolecules at a time, a parallel approach can be attempted; genomics and proteomics are some technologies used in this process. Secretomics has also emerged as an important technology in the high-throughput search for biomarkers; however, significant technical difficulties remain. Although all the primary biomarkers – carbohydrates, nucleic acids, proteins and lipids can serve as biomarkers but proteins are preferred and superior, due to dynamic nature of protein profile over time and space.

- Spingomylins
- Gangliosides
- Cerebrosides
- Many more...

- Glucose (For diabetes)
- Glycoprotein (for blood type)
- Many More...

Lipids   **Sugars**

Biomarkers

Proteins   **Nucleic acids**

- Insulin
- P53
- Many more...

- SNPs
- CNVs
- RFLP
- Many more....

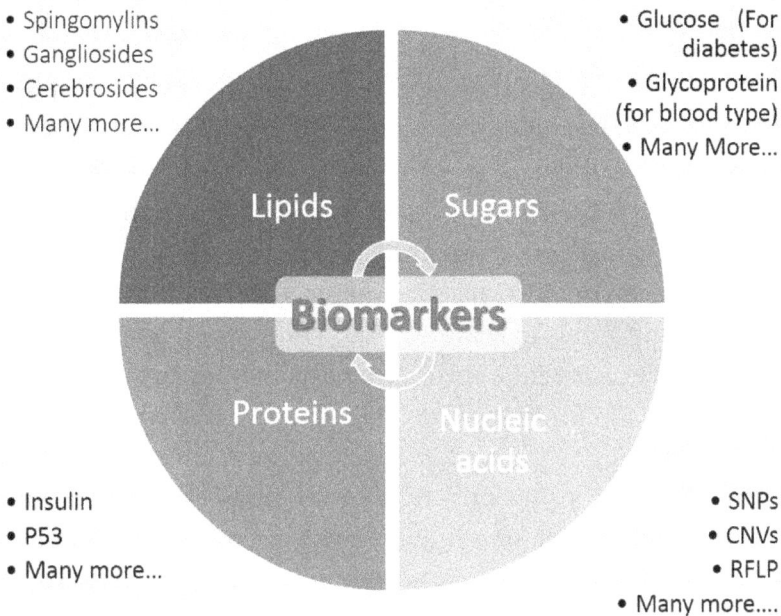

Figure 3.6: Four basic biomolecules are preferred biomarkers for most of the pathological conditions (SNPs – Single nucleotide polymorphism; CNVs – copy number variations; RFLP – restriction fragment length polymorphism).

The identification of clinically significant protein biomarkers of phenotype and biological function is an expanding area of research which will extend diagnostic capabilities. Biomarkers for a number of diseases have recently emerged, including prostate specific antigen (PSA) for prostate cancer [92] and C-reactive protein (CRP) for heart disease[93]. The epigenetic clock which measures the age of cells/tissues/organs based on DNA methylation levels is arguably the most accurate genomic biomarker. Using biomarkers from easily assessable biofluids (e.g. blood and urine) is beneficial in evaluating the state of harder-to-reach tissues and organs. Biofluids are more readily accessible, unlike more invasive or unfeasible techniques (such as tissue biopsy).

Biofluids contain proteins from tissues and serve as effective hormonal communicators. The tissue acts as a transmitter of information, and the biofluid (sampled by physician) acts as a receiver. The informativeness of the biofluid relies on the fidelity of the channel. Sources of noise which decrease fidelity include the addition of proteins derived from other tissues (or from the biofluid itself); proteins may also be lost through glomerular filtration[94]. These factors can significantly influence the protein composition of a biofluid[95]. In addition, simply looking at protein overlap would miss information transmission occurring through classes of proteins and protein-protein interactions.

Instead, the proteins' projection onto functional, drug, and disease spaces allow measurement of the functional distance between tissue and biofluids. Proximity in these abstract spaces signifies a low level of distortion across the information channel (and, hence, high performance by the biofluid). However, current approaches to biomarker prediction have analyzed tissues and biofluids separately. Conventional method to determine and discover proteomic biomarker involves the use of global proteomics techniques. Classical proteomic techniques such as two-dimetional gel electrophoresis and silver staining followed by MALDI-TOF based analysis has now become obsolete and newer technologies such as quantitative or semi-quantitative analysis of proteins using high throughput techniques such as iTRAQ, SiLAC, iCAT etc is now gaining attention. Newer platforms involving electrospray ionization techniques and detection using quadrupole are becoming preferred choice for biomarker discovery in proteomics. Antibody array and tissue microarray are emerging technique that would enable large scale screening and validation of putative biomarkers. Unlike conventional scientific experiments, biomarker discovery involves screening of very large number of samples with inclusion of samples from different ethnicity, regions and genetic makeup. Epigenetic factors such as environment, diet etc. are also included to consider the evaluation of a protein as biomarker. Therefore, despite of the technological advancements, the biomarker discovery remains a challenge and the ratio of potential candidate biomarker (putative biomarkers) and established biomarkers is very low.

3.4   Quantitative Proteomics: A High Throughput Tool

Quantitative proteomics is an emerging domain of proteomics that includes approaches used for both discovery and understanding global proteomic dynamics in a cell, tissue or organism. Most quantitative proteomic analyses utilize the isotopic labeling of proteins or peptides in the experimental groups, which can then be differentiated by mass spectrometry.

Relative quantitation methods (SILAC, ICAT, ICPL and isobaric tags) are used to compare protein or peptide abundance between samples, while spiking unlabeled samples with known concentrations of isotopically labeled synthetic peptides can yield absolute quantitation of target peptides (via SRM). Label-free strategies are also available for both relative and absolute quantitation. Although these strategies are more complex than mere protein identification, quantitative proteomics is critical for our understanding global protein expression and modifications underlying the molecular mechanisms of biological processes and disease states. In the following section a detailed description of quantitative proteomics is provided with recent report on hypoxia research showing the use of quantitative proteomics.

Early biochemical proteomics research focused on identifying and understanding the functions of individual proteins or protein complexes. Technological advances in instrumentation, have increased the number of proteins that one can analyze in a single sample from hundreds a decade ago to thousands today.[96] At this level of analysis, global protein dynamics can be studied on a cellular, tissue or organism level. This type of approach is consistent with the increasingly broad-scope analyses that are being used in other life science fields, including genomics, transcriptomics, metabolomics, and kinemics, to give us a greater understanding of global biological processes and how they respond to different stimuli or change during disease states. While proteomic analyses can be used to qualitatively identify thousands of proteins in cells or other biological samples, there is also a need to quantitate these proteins. Because of the dynamic and interactive nature of proteins, though, quantitative proteomics is considerably more complex than simply identifying proteins in a sample. But due of the considerable amount of data that one can acquire from quantitative proteomics, this approach is critical for our understanding global protein kinetics and molecular mechanisms of biological processes.

Two fundamental approaches to proteomic analyses are currently employed. In top-down proteomics, intact proteins or large fragments are ionized and analyzed by mass spectrometry (MS). Bottom-up proteomics rely on peptides, which are generated by proteolytic digestion of protein samples. Due to the protein size limitation in top-down proteomics (< 50kD), bottom-up proteomics is more commonly used. Because of the overwhelming number of proteotypic peptides in a sample, only a small subset of all peptides in a sample can be analyzed in a single MS run, which limits the number of proteins in a sample that can be identified. The number of proteins available for quantitation is further limited, because they have to be identified in all samples that are tested in a single experiment. Practically speaking, the linear dynamic range of quantitation is often limited to 10- to 20-fold, depending on the sensitivity of the instrument and complexity of the sample, which also affects the scope of quantitative proteomics.

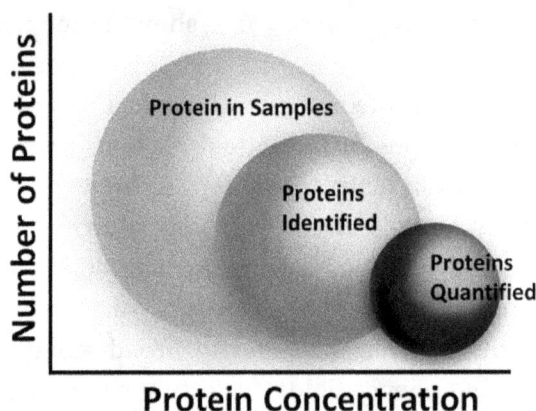

Figure 3.7: Protein availability for quantitative proteomic analysis is limited. Protein abundance and sample complexity are significant factors that affect the availability of proteins for mass spectrometric quantitation (Redrawn after Bantscheff et al.)[97]

Sample complexity is a critical factor of peptide quantitation, as identification and quantification rates are directly proportional to sample complexity. Methods such as affinity purification are often performed to remove high-abundance proteins and reduce sample complexity. In-line liquid chromatography (LC) is also a common Pre-MS Fractionation process to chemically separate peptides to further reduce sample complexity. Quantitative proteomic analyses typically rely on MS to identify or quantitate selected peptides, although tandem mass spectrometry (MS/MS) is required for peptide identification. During the first round of MS (MS1), ionized peptides are sampled to produce a precursor ion spectrum that represents all ionized peptides in the sample. Individual ions are then selected to undergo collision-induced fragmentation (CID) and a second round of MS (MS2), which yields a fragment ion spectrum for each precursor ion. These fragment spectra are compared to peptide databases and assigned specific peptide sequences and then computationally organized into the predicted protein sequence.

3.4.1   Relative vs. Absolute Quantitation

Mass spectrometry is not inherently quantitative, because proteolytic peptides show great variability in physiochemical properties that in turn result in variability in mass spectrometric response between runs. Additionally, mass spectrometers only sample a small percentage of the total peptides in a sample[97]. Therefore, various approaches have been developed to perform relative and absolute proteomic quantitation. Relative quantitation strategies compare the levels of individual peptides in a sample to those in an identical, but experimentally modified, sample. One approach for relative quantitation is to separately analyzing samples by MS and compare the spectra to determine peptide abundance in one sample relative to another, as in label-free quantitation strategies.

More costly and time-consuming approaches require internal, isotopically labeled standards for the mass spectrometer to distinguish between identical proteins from separate samples. A typical relative quantitation experiment that uses isotopic labels entails labeling proteins or peptides from two experimental samples with isotopically heavy and light atoms (via a labeled amino acid or cell culture component), which makes the peptides in these two samples isotopologues (identical molecules that differ only in isotope composition). After alteration of the proteome in the experimental group through chemical treatment or genetic manipulation, equal amounts of protein from both populations are combined and analyzed by LC-MS or LC-MS/MS analysis. Because the light and heavy forms of individual peptides are chemically identical, they co-elute during LC pre-fractionation and are therefore detected simultaneously during MS analysis. The peak intensities of the heavy and light peptides are then compared to determine the change in abundance in one sample relative to that of the other sample. Methods to isotopically label proteins or peptides include metabolic labeling of live cells and enzymatic or chemical labeling of extracted proteins or peptides.

Absolute proteomic quantitation using isotopic peptides entails spiking known concentrations of synthetic, heavy isotopologues of target peptides into an experimental sample and then performing LC-MS/MS. As with relative quantitation using isotopic labels, peptides of equal chemistry co-elute and are analyzed by MS simultaneously. Unlike relative quantitation, though, the abundance of the target peptide in the experimental sample is compared to that of the heavy peptide and back-calculated to the initial concentration of the standard using a pre-determined standard curve to yield the absolute quantitation of the target peptide.

It may seem obvious that absolute quantitation would be ideal compared to relative quantitation, because the absolute peptide values from different samples could also be compared to determine relative protein changes. Relative proteomic quantitation is used more often than absolute quantitation, though, because costly reagents and time-consuming assay development are required for the absolute quantitation of each protein of interest.

Experimental bias can influence the decision to use relative or absolute quantitation strategies. One source of bias is the mass spectrometer itself, which has a limited capacity to detect low-abundance peptides in samples with a high dynamic range. Additionally, the limited duty cycle of mass spectrometers restricts the number of collisions per unit of time, which may result in an undersampling of complex proteomic samples[98]. Another source of bias is variation in sample preparation between experiments or individual samples in single experiments. The greater the number of steps between labeling and sample combination, the greater is the risk of introducing experimental bias. For example, during metabolic labeling, proteins are labeled in live animals or cells and the samples are then immediately combined. Because all subsequent sample preparation and analysis is performed with the combined samples, metabolic labeling has the lowest risk of experimental variation[97]. Conversely, samples that are individually processed and analyzed in label-free quantitation strategies have a greater risk of sample variation and experimental bias.

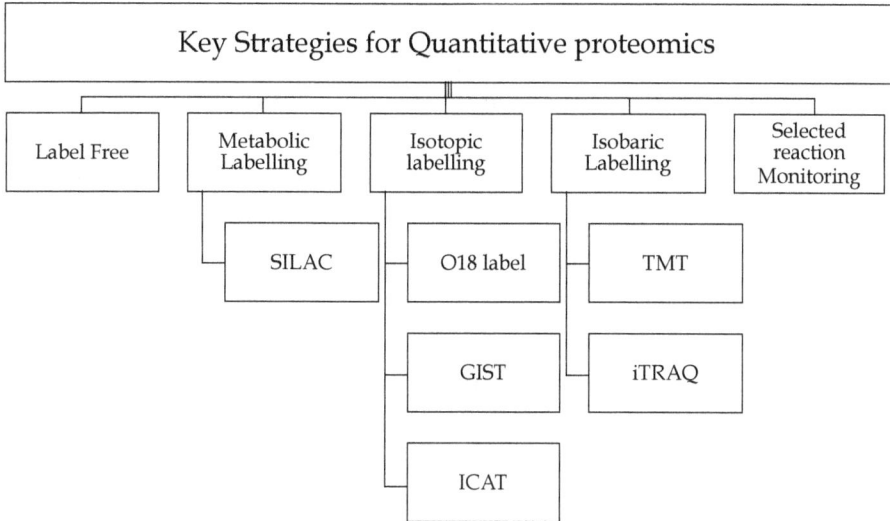

Figure 3.3: Various strategies for quantitative proteomics.

3.4.2   Label free Quantitation

Label-free methods for both relative and absolute quantitation have been developed as a rapid and low-cost alternative to other quantitative proteomic approaches. These strategies are ideal for large-sample analyses in clinical screening or biomarker discovery experiments[99], and while they are good at measuring large changes in protein expression, they are less reliable for measuring small changes and can have a limited range of linear quantitative measurement (< 2 orders of magnitude)[100].

Unlike other quantitation methods, label-free samples are separately collected, prepared and analyzed by LC-MS or LC-MS/MS. Because of this, label-free quantitation experiments need to be more carefully controlled than stable isotope methods to account for any experimental variations. Protein quantitation is performed using either ion peak intensity or spectral counting.

Relative quantitation by ion peak intensity relies on LC-MS only (no MS/MS). The direct MS m/z values for all ions are detected and their signal intensities at a particular time recorded. The signal intensity from electrospray ionization has been reported to highly correlate with ion concentration, and therefore the relative peptide levels between samples can be determined directly from these peak intensities[101,102]. Because of the large amount of data collected from these experiments, sensitive computer algorithms are required for automated ion peak alignment and comparison.

Label-free relative quantitation by spectral counts entails comparing the sum of the MS/MS spectra from a given peptide across multiple samples, which has been shown to directly correlate with protein abundance[101]. Unlike quantitation by peak intensity, spectral counting does not require special algorithms or other tools, although significant normalization is required[103,104].

Besides relative quantitation, label-free methods can be used to determine the absolute concentration of proteins in a sample. One method entails determining the exponentially modified protein abundance index (emPAI), which estimates protein abundance based on the number of peptides detected and the number of theoretically observed tryptic peptides for each protein, is used to determine the approximate absolute protein abundance in large-scale proteomic analyses[99]. Another method, absolute protein expression (APEX), is based on spectral counts and uses correction factors to make protein abundance proportional to the number of peptides observed.

3.4.3   Metabolic Labelling or SILAC

Metabolic labeling for relative proteomic quantitation was first reported by Oda *et al.*, who uniformly labeled all amino acids in yeast with heavy nitrogen (15N) by growing yeast in culture medium where the only nitrogen source was 15N-labeled ammonium persulfate[105]. This approach was further developed for use in mammalian cell lines by Mann *et al.*, who reported a method for stable isotope labeling by amino acids in cell culture (SILAC), which has become the most common approach for in vivo isotopic labeling[106]. Instead of labeling all amino acids with heavy nitrogen, cells are cultured in growth medium that contains 13C6-lysine and/or 13C6-arginine. These amino acids were chosen, because trypsin, the predominant enzyme used to generate proteotypic peptides for MS analysis, cleaves at the C-terminus of lysine and arginine. Thus, all tryptic peptides from cultures grown in SILAC media (except for the very C-terminal peptides) have at least one labeled amino acid, which results in a constant mass increment in labeled samples over non-labeled, yet otherwise identical, samples.

There are many benefits of using metabolic labeling strategies compared to other methods of quantitation. For one, proteins can often attain >90% isotopic incorporation in immortalized cell lines after 6-8 passages[106]. Because heavy and light samples are combined before sample preparation for MS analysis, the level of quantitation bias from processing errors is low. This key aspect of metabolic labeling makes this method particularly useful to detect relatively small changes in protein levels or post-translational modifications between experimental conditions.

3.4.4   Isotopic Tags

For samples that are not amenable to metabolic labeling, such as when analyzing clinical samples (e.g., biological fluids, tissue samples) or when experimental time is limited, chemical or enzymatic stable isotopic labeling methods are available for quantitative proteomic analyses. These include strategies to add isotopic atoms or isotope-coded tags to peptides or proteins. While the methods described below do not comprise an exhaustive list of isotopic labeling methods, they do represent commonly used approaches.

Enzymatic labeling with 18O takes advantage of the proteolytic mechanism of trypsin to incorporate two heavy oxygen atoms from $H_2 18O$ at the C-terminus of every newly digested peptide[107]. In this labeling scheme, one sample is digested with trypsin and18O water and another with 16O water, and then the samples are combined for relative proteomic analysis by MS. While this method is simple to execute, a disadvantage is a slow back exchange of 18O and 16O when the two samples are combined, leading to incomplete labeling or peptides labeled with only one heavy oxygen atom. While adding 1-5% formic acid can attenuate this back exchange for up to 24 hours, samples labeled with this method should be processed rapidly[108].

Another enzymatic isotopic labeling strategy is global internal standard technology (GIST), which uses deuterated (2H) acylating agents such as N-acetoxysuccinimide (NAS) to label primary amino groups on digested peptides[109]. Acylation of these groups, though, changes the ionic states of peptides and may affect the ionization efficiency of peptides with C-terminal lysines[110]. Additionally, isotopic methods that label with deuterium result in partial separation of heavy and light peptides during LC, because the deuterium slightly interacts with the stationary phase (e.g., C18). This difference can affect the confidence and accuracy of the internal standards, because one of them may co-elute with another peptide that inhibits its ionization.

A rapid and relatively inexpensive method of chemical labeling is stable isotope dimethylation. This approach uses formaldehyde in deuterated water to label primary amines with deuterated methyl groups[110]. Unlike GIST, this approach does not change the ionic state of the labeled peptides because of the reductive amination that occurs, so their chemical properties remain the same as those of unlabeled peptides.

A benefit of this approach is that a wide array of sample types is amenable to formaldehyde fixation, which is fast and cheap compared to other labeling reagents. As with other methods of labeling, this method has global labeling characteristics, which has both pros and cons. While this high level of isotopic labeling is beneficial when other labeling strategies fail, it requires either using relative pure samples or sample preparation to reduce the complexity of biological samples to minimize the number of peaks detected by MS. Commercially isotopic labeling reagents are also available that encompass a wide range of reactive groups for different crosslinker specificity and heavy labels for different applications isotopologue separation.

The isotope-coded affinity tag (ICAT) method was developed to reduce the sample complexity and identify low-abundance proteins and peptides in complex samples[111]. ICAT tags were originally comprised of a sulfhydryl-reactive chemical crosslinking group, an 8-fold deuterated (d8; adds 8 Da to the molecular mass of the unlabeled peptide) or light (d0) linker region and a biotin molecule. Because of the sulfhydryl-reactive chemical group, only free thiols on cysteine residues are labeled with this tag. The sample is then passed over immobilized avidin, which binds to the biotin tag and purifies the labeled peptides from the sample. Because not all peptides have cysteine residues, this method does not result in global labeling and thus is an inherent approach to reduce sample complexity. Once peptides are labeled, they are eluted from the sample by column chromatography using immobilized avidin or streptavidin. After purification, heavy (d8) and light (d0) samples are combined and analyzed for relative quantitation by LC-MS.

3.4.5   Isobaric Tags

Unlike isotopic tags that have the potential to separate during LC elution, isobaric tags have identical masses and chemical properties that allow heavy and light isotopologues to co-elute together. The tags are then cleaved from the peptides by collision-induced dissociation (CID) during MS/MS, which is required for this type of quantitative proteomic analysis. Indeed, these tags were originally called tandem mass tags to indicate their use with tandem mass spectrometry[112]. After CID, the peptide fragment ions are analyzed for sequence assignment and the isobaric tags are quantitated, resulting in concurrent peptide identification and relative quantitation. Additionally, because MS/MS is required to detect the isobaric tags, unlabeled peptides are not quantitated.

A benefit of isobaric mass tags is the multiplex capabilities and thus increased throughput potential of this approach. Commercially available isobaric mass tags (e.g., TMT*, iTRAQ*) are commercially available that offer the simultaneously analysis of 4, 6 or 8 biological samples. While the exact tags used vary depending on manufacturer, the basic components of all isobaric mass tag reagents consist of a mass reporter (tag) that has a unique number of 13C substitutions, a mass normalizer that has a unique mass that balances the mass of the tag to make all of the tags equal in mass. Isobaric mass tags also have a reactive moiety that crosslinks to primary amines or cysteines (depending on the product used). These tags are designed so that the mass tag is cleaved at a specific linker region upon high-energy CID (HCD), yielding the different-sized tags that are then quantitated by LC-MS/MS. Isobaric mass tagging has also been adapted for use with protein labeling (similar to ICPL). Some commercially available kits also offer isobaric tags with sulfhydryl-reactivity and anti-TMT antibody for affinity purification of cysteine-tagged peptides prior to LC-MS/MS.

3.4.6   Selected Reaction Monitoring (SRM) and Targeted Assay Development

Selected reaction monitoring (SRM) or multiple reaction monitoring (MRM) is a method of absolute quantitation (also terms AQUA) in targeted proteomics analyses that is performed by spiking complex samples with stable isotope-labeled synthetic peptides that act as internal standards for specific peptides[113]. These heavy peptides are designed to be identical to tryptic

Method	Dynamic range	Coverage	Quant accuracy, (throughput) R = relative A = absolute
Label-free			
2D gels	1 to 4 stain dependent	Medium	Medium (low). R. Requires MS identification.
Ion intensities MS[1]	3	Good	Medium (medium to high). R. LC dependent.
Spectrum count MS[2]	3 Inaccurate for low abundance.	Good	Poor (medium to high). R. LC dependent
APEX,emPAI	3 or 4	Good	Poor (high). R. Within sample only.
Metabolic labeling			
^{15}N	1 to 2	Medium	Precise (low). R. Between 2 conditions.
SILAC	1 to 2	Medium	Precise (low). R. Between 2 and 3 samples.
Isotopic labeling			
ICAT, ^{18}O, ICPL	1 to 2	Poor	Precise (low). R. Between 2 conditions.
Isobaric labeling			
ITRAQ, TMT, DIGE	2 3	Medium	Medium (low). R or A. Between 2 and 8 conditions.
Targeted			
MRM Isotope dilution +/– heavy label	5 Attomolar detection.	Poor	Precise (high). R or A. Requires intensive method development.

Table 1: Overview of the main approaches for quantitative proteomics. Modified from Wasinger et al.[115]

peptides generated by sample digestion, so that they co-elute with the target peptide and are concomitantly analyzed by MS/MS (using instrumentation with a large dynamic range). The target peptide concentration is then determined by measuring the observed signal response for the target peptide relative to that of the heavy peptide, the concentration of which is calculated from a pre-determined calibration-response curve. While this method yields absolute peptide concentrations in as few as one sample, calibration curves have to be generated for each target peptide in the sample.

Assay development is a significant part of SRM proteomic analyses. Heavy peptides for each of the target peptides must be synthesized, and because proteins yield multiple peptides with varying electrochemical characteristics, the heavy peptide sequences that will yield the optimal results must be identified. Software is used to help predict the ideal tryptic peptide sequences, but the combination of trial-and-error peptide identification and instrumentation optimization makes absolute quantitation using isotopic peptides time-consuming and costly. Once the assay is optimized for a predetermined set of peptides (up to approx. 200 per LC-MS run; 15), though, SRM offers the highest level of reproducibility and sensitivity in detecting these peptides in multiple samples. This approach has been reported to detect proteins with concentrations less than 50 copies per cell in unfractionated lysates [114], demonstrating that it is the quantitative approach that is the least affected by sample complexity[96].

AQUA-grade peptides are costly because of their high quality and purity, and therefore scientists often use low-quality crude peptides during targeted assay development. Entire libraries of different peptide sequences can be commercially synthesized and screened during assay development to identify the optimum peptides, which are then synthesized at the AQUA purity and quality standards for SRM assays.

3.4.7   Quantitative Proteomics in Hypobaric-hypoxia Studies Remains Poetically Unexplored

Till date, not many studies on hypobaric hypoxia have been performed using quantitative proteomics. However, among only very studies that have been done show a remarkable difference in the conclusions drawn from classical studies and therefore suggest the extreme potentials of quantitative proteomics in biomarker discovery of high altitude associated pathophysiology. Among such studies one that was performed by Julian *et al.* in 2013 showed that after 9 hours of hypoxia the abundance of proteins with antioxidant properties (i.e., peroxiredoxin 6, glutathione peroxidase and sulfhydryl oxidase 1) rose in AMS but not AMS•R. Their exploratory analyses suggested that exposure to hypobaric hypoxia enhances enzymatic antioxidant systems in AMS vs. AMS•R which, they propose, may be an overcompensation for hypoxia-induced oxidant production. And therefor it was speculated that quenching oxidant activity may have adverse downstream effects that are of pathophysiological importance for AMS such as interrupting oxidant-sensitive cell signaling and gene transcription, and 2) question the existing assumption that increased oxidant production in AMS is pathological. In this study plasma samples were pooled according to AMS status at each time point. Protein composition of the samples was determined by a GeLC-MS/MS approach using two analytical platforms (LTQ-XL Linear Ion Trap Mass Spectrometer and a LTQ-FT Ultra Hybrid Mass Spectrometer) for technical replication. Spectral counting was used to make semi-quantitative comparisons of protein abundance between AMS-susceptible (AMS) and AMS-resistant (AMS•R) subjects with exposure to hypobaric hypoxia. No other exclusive study on hypobaric hypoxia based on quantitative proteomics could be retrieved from popular bibilometric databases suggesting a wide scope of this domain to re-explore the protein expression profiles at a high throughput scale.

3.5   Bioinformatics Insight into Hypobaric-hypoxia Proteomics

Computational biology plays a significant role in the discovery of new biomarkers, the analyses of disease states and the validation of potential biomarkers. Biomarkers are used to measure the progress of disease or the physiological effects of therapeutic intervention in the treatment of disease. Biomarkers are also used as early warning signs for various diseases such as cancer and inflammatory diseases. Bioinformatics approaches are critical for effectively mining high-dimensional data to provide insights into disease biology. Data preprocessing such as background correction and spectrum alignment are critical issues before data mining. High dimensional data needs to be reduced to fewer variables using feature selection.

Many algorithms exist to mine large datasets, but no specific approach is ideal or applicable to all study designs. For data mining, best approach would be to utilize feature selection algorithm with cross validation. It is better to utilize different approaches in parallel to arrive at a final algorithm. With increasing availability of public data, rigorous comparisons of data preprocessing and data mining approaches are needed. Most of the proteomics studies are performed on small populations. It is possible that small sample size may result in potential biomarkers failing the validation test. MS is increasingly being used to analyze complex protein mixtures to recognize biomarker patterns. SELDI based profiling appears to successfully detect some previously unknown proteins. Also, there is evidence that biomarker patterns can be found that can differentiate cancerous and normal individuals. Finally, it is anticipated that existing and emerging computational data mining approaches along with rigorous and systematic evaluation, will help to unleash the full biological potential of proteomic profiling.

3.5.1   Data Mining

Data-points obtained from the data preprocessing step represent potential biomarkers. Many profiling studies aim to find proteomic patterns that can discriminate between different biological conditions. In order to properly assign statistical significance to candidate biomarkers, or any changes in apparent protein abundance, it is important to understand the patterns of variability. Before subjecting the data to data mining algorithms, a feature selection step is used which can be performed on raw data or the detected peaks using unsupervised learning approaches (approaches do not take into account class labels; analogous to clustering) or supervised learning approaches (approaches accounts for class labels; analogous to classification) which are discussed below. Yu et.al implemented a random forest algorithm to find markers that can best discriminate cases from control sample[116,117]. Pratapa et.al compared feature selection with Fisher discriminant ratio (FDR), followed by classification accuracy of a linear SVM versus joint feature selection and classification with Bayesian sparse multinomial logistic regression (SMLR). The SMLR approach outperformed FDR and SVM, but both were effective in achieving good diagnostic accuracy with a small number of features [118]. Once the features are selected, the data undergoes transformation due to high variance in a given input variable.

3.5.2   Normalization

The normalization step helps to reduce variation due to experimental noise from systemic effect between samples, e.g., from varying amounts of applied protein, degradation over time in the sample, or change in the column or sensitivity of instrument. Normalization of MS data can be performed either by coercing the *m/z* intensity values to be comparable across experiments (low level processing), or by altering the peak abundance to be comparable (mid-level processing). In general, one aims to normalize not only replicates, but also experimental data of distinct biological origin, such as serum profiles from cancer patients and healthy case controls. The underlying assumption behind normalization is that the overall MS abundance of all features (peaks or time-*m/z* pairs), or subset(s) of these, should be equal across different experiments[119]. Global normalization refers to cases where all features are simultaneously used to determine a single normalization factor between two experiments, while local normalization refers to cases where a subset of features are used at a time (different subsets for different parts of the data). A global normalization is followed by a probability model to investigate the intensity dependent missing events and provides possible substitutions for the missing values [120].

3.5.3   Some Studies on Hypobaric-hypoxia using Classical Bioinformatics Approaches

As we have seen above, the most common usage of Bioinformatics and computational biology in the biomarker discovery lies in the data mining, especially to match the experimental spectral peaks and to perform the data normalization. Yet some of the other interesting features of the hypoxia dynamics that remain unexplored are the study of protein dynamics in hypoxic conditions. Many of the previous studies on polymorphisms have shown that small alterations in the basic amino acids sequence of protein leads to minor conformational changes but they are more pronounced in terms the protein activity. These effects are closely related and accountable for the difference in susceptibility of individuals to high altitude. Some of the naïve attempts have been however made to validate the use conventional prophylaxis and in silico evaluation of candidate drug molecules.

In a study done by David *et al.*, authors showed that the interaction of bacoside-TPH complex using three different docking algorithms such as HexDock, PatchDock and AutoDock. All these three algorithms showed that bacoside A and A3 well fit into the cavity consists of active sites[121]. Further, our analysis revealed that major active compounds bacoside A3 and A interact with different residues of TPH through hydrogen bond. Interestingly, Tyr235, Thr265 and Glu317 are the key residues among them, but none of them are either at tryptophan or BH4 binding region. However, it's noteworthy to mention that Tyr 235 is a catalytic sensitive residue, Thr265 is present in the flexible loop region and Glu317 is known to interact with Fe. Interactions with these residues may critically regulate TPH function and thus serotonin synthesis. Our study suggested that the interaction of bacosides (A3/A) with TPH might up-regulate its activity to elevate the biosynthesis of 5-HT, thereby enhances learning and memory formation. In another study by Saraswat *et al.*, authors identification some of the novel candidate molecules that block VEGF-A site using in silico approaches. In this study, the active site residues of VEGF-A were detected by Pocketfinder, CASTp, and DogSiteScorer. Based on in silico data, three VEGF-A blocker (VAB) candidate molecules (VAB1, VAB2, and VAB3) were checked for improvement in cellular viability and regulation of VEGF levels in N2a cells under hypoxia (0.5% O_2). Additionally, the best candidate molecule's efficacy was assessed in male Sprague-Dawley rats for its ameliorative effect on cerebral oedema and vascular leakage under hypobaric hypoxia equivalent to 7260 m was determined[122]. All experimental results were compared with the commercially available VEGF blocker sunitinib. Vascular endothelial growth factor-A blocker 1 was found most effective in increasing cellular viability and maintaining normal VEGF levels under hypoxia (0.5% oxygen) in N2a cells. Vascular endothelial growth factor-A blocker 1 effectively restored VEGF levels, decreased cerebral oedema, and reduced vascular leakage under hypobaric hypoxia when compared to sunitinib-treated rats. Vascular endothelial growth factor-A blocker 1 may be a promising candidate molecule for ameliorating hypobaric hypoxia-induced vasogenic oedema by regulating VEGF levels[123].

4

Proteins Biomarkers for Hypoxia: Quest is On

Given the scale and challenges of hypobaric hypoxia (as described in chapter 1 and 2) the scientific attention is more towards solving the clinical or preclinical question especially to develop finer methods for diagnosis and discovery of molecules suitable as disease targets. Identification of Protein biomarkers for the hypoxia was once the biggest challenge when the initial studies on hypobaric-hypoxia were undertaken during early 1970s. With the advent of technologies and progressive addition of information on proteomic and genomic changes during the hypobaric hypoxia the quest became easier. As described in the previous chapter a biomarker should be unique and consistent across the population, which means a large number of samples needed to be screened before confirming the biomarker status of a protein. The need of biomarker discovery is primarily to enable the early diagnosis and therapeutic targets.

4.1   Optimization of Method for Proteomic Analysis of Human Plasma

Proteome analysis of plasma is increasingly leading to biomarker discovery of human diseases. However the highly abundant proteins, excess of salt and lipid in plasma makes the analysis very challenging. Therefore it is necessary to improve the sample preparation procedures before/after the two-dimensional gel electrophoresis analysis of plasma proteins and this was considered as the primary objective during the initial years of biomarker discovery on hypobaric hypoxia at author's lab. The objective of study was to develop a reproducible method by examining the following parameters:

a. Depletion of the high-abundant proteins

b. Effect of different precipitation methods

c. Comparing optimized rehydration buffer using modified Taguchi method and

d. comparing the effects of different staining methods.

Our results showed that the depletion of two high-abundant proteins improved the visualization of less abundant proteins present in human plasma and precipitation with TCA/acetone resulted in an efficient sample concentration and desalting. We found that using optimized rehydration buffer as compared to standard rehydration buffer increased protein solubility, improved resolution and reproducibility of 2D gels. We also found that visualization of 2D gel profiles by silver staining and fluorescent staining enhanced the detection of low abundant plasma proteins as compared to Coomassie staining. In conclusion, the optimized conditions in our study can be applied to produce a better reference 2-DE gel of plasma samples for the identification of novel disease markers. Also, it is very important to deplete the high abundance proteins such as albumin and serum immunoglobulins which predominate the plasma proteins and likely to mask the low abundant proteins. This is usually performed using conventional kits and methods. The level of depletion is often checked using 1DGE and coommasie staining before further analysis of proteins (Figure 4.1).

In order to use the information rich proteomic analysis of plasma in a diagnostic manner, it is essential that the method used to prepare the sample provide reproducible results. Although a variety of proteomic techniques have been attempted so far, no generally applicable technique has yet been developed for the identification of biomarker that can replace 2-DE with regard to its ability to separate and display several thousand plasma proteins simultaneously. The selection of an appropriate blood plasma preparation method is important for confident 2-DE results. The goal of the present study was to find the optimized method for a high throughout sample analysis of human plasma by 2-DE.

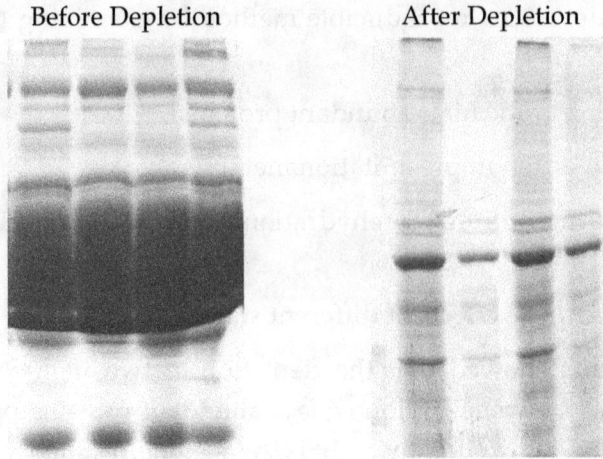

Figure 4.1: Coommasie stained 1D gels: these gels are generally prepared to test the level of depletion of abundant proteins before carrying out further 2D gele electrophoresis analysis

The use of plasma as a protein sample because a large number of plasma samples are usually analyzed for diagnostic purposes and marker detection. This work describes that the selection and use of anticoagulants and protease inhibitors during blood collection increases the chances for consistent results. The removal of highly abundant proteins using an albumin and IgG removal kit results in 4- to 6- fold increase in relative protein concentration of medium- and low- abundance proteins . As a result, the detection, identification and quantification of medium and low- abundance human plasma proteins by proteomic methods should easily achieved and aid in the characterization of the important human plasma proteome. TCA/acetone precipitation improves the pattern generated during 2-DE. The contribution of different detergents in the rehydration solution improves the solubility and resolution of proteins on 2D gels. The staining profile of proteins with the most sensitive method improves the detection of low abundance proteins in plasma. In conclusion, our study suggests that by using these procedures/steps for sample preparation before and after 2-DE analysis one can increase the likelihood of discovery of biomarkers of high sensitivity and specificity that can be used in early disease detection, as well as to monitor disease progression. Readers are advised to read the complete study at http://www.omicsonline.org/

analysis-of-human-plasma-proteome-using-two-dimensional-gel-electroph
oresis-jpb.1000111.php?aid=1415.[124]

4.2   Protein Biomarkers for Hypobaric Hypoxia using Rat Model

Once the optimization was completed, we began our quest for biomarkers for hyporic hypoxia induced pathophysiological changes. Initial studies were planned using experimental rat model of hypobaric hypoxia using simulated hypoxia in custom designed hypoxia chambers. In this study we investigated the temporal plasma protein alterations of rat induced by hypobaric hypoxia at a simulated altitude of 7620 m (25,000 ft, 282 mm Hg) in a hypobaric chamber. Total plasma proteins collected at different time points (0, 6, 12 and 24 h), separated by two-dimensional electrophoresis (2-DE) and identified using matrix assisted laser desorption ionization time of flight (MALDI-TOF/TOF). Biological processes that were enriched in the plasma proteins during hypobaric hypoxia were identified using Gene Ontology (GO) analysis. According to their properties and obvious alterations during hypobaric hypoxia, changes of plasma concentrations of Ttr, Prdx-2, Gpx -3, Apo A-I, Hp, Apo-E, Fetub and Nme were selected to be validated by Western blot analysis.

To our knowledge, this was the first comprehensive proteome study reporting the proteome level changes in plasma of rats exposed to acute hypobaric hypoxia. Our results obtained by 2-DE electrophoresis and partly also confirmed by the use of other techniques, indicate that short-term acute hypobaric hypoxia not only identify hypoxia-modulated early proteins but also altered distinct biological process depending on the stress duration. The relationships of these proteins with hypobaric hypoxia are elucidated in the following section.

In this study, three cellular antioxidants, thioredoxin domain containing protein 12, peroxiredoxin-2 and glutathione peroxidase 3 were identified in the plasma of rats treated with hypobaric hypoxia. Thioredoxin domain containing protein 12 (TXNDC12) belongs to the thioredoxin super family. Members of this super family possess a thioredoxin fold with a consensus active site sequence (CxxC) and have roles in redox regulation, defense against oxidative stress, refolding of disulfide-containing proteins, and regulation of transcription factors.[125] In this study, TXNDC12 was up-regulated, suggesting the protective of TXNDC in the cellular defense against oxidative stress caused by hypobaric hypoxia. Peroxiredoxins (PRDXS) are H_2O_2 scavenging antioxidant proteins and six mammalian isoforms (I– VI) have been identified. They are small proteins (22–27 kDa) and all have the common thioredoxin CxxC motif and catalyze peroxide detoxification.[101] Increased expression of different peroxiredoxins has been reported in lung cancer, alveolitis, and hypoxic conditions[126]. Peroxiredoxin-2 (PRDX2) belongs to a ubiquitous PRX family, which has been shown to have multiple functions such as enhancing natural killer cell activity[127] increasing cell resistance to oxidative stress[128], regulating transcription activator protein[129] protecting erythrocytes against oxidative stress[130], and anti- HIV activity[131]. In light of its multifaceted biological functions, the increased plasma level of PRDX2 might play a multifunctional role during the acute inflammation induced by hypobaric hypoxia. Glutathione peroxidase 3 (GPX-3) functions in response to oxidative damage by catalyzing the reduction of hydrogen peroxide, lipid peroxides, and organic hydroperoxide. Rousseau *et al.* reported the increase in plasma glutathione peroxidase activity as a potential indicator of hypoxic stress in breath-hold diving[132]. Interestingly recent study from our group showed that 'hypoxia sensitive' animals fail to increase GPX3 after acute hypobaric hypoxia[133]. Despite significant difference in experimental conditions employed in these two studies (exposure time and altitude), it is likely that the upregulation of GPX-3 could play a role in acclimatization to hypobaric hypoxia. Sulfonate conjugation is an important pathway in the metabolism of a variety of endogenous and exogenous compounds, including estrogens and other mammary carcinogens. This reaction is catalyzed by SULTs, 3 a superfamily of multifunctional enzymes including six cytosolic SULTs that have been identified in human tissues. Sulfotransferase 1A1 (SULT 1A, spot no: 23) is one of the most important members in this enzyme family due to its extensive tissue distribution and abundance. This enzyme has a substantially higher activity than other SULTs in catalyzing the sulfonation of 4-nitrophenol, a commonly used assay in biochemical pharmacogenetic studies for testing the activity of thermostable phenol SULTs.[134] SULT1A1 catalyzes the sulfonation of estrogens to form water-soluble and biologically inactive estrogen sulfates, reducing the level of estrogen exposure in their target tissues.[135] The mutation in the SULT1A1 gene would affect an individual's capacity to efficiently sulfate endogenous compounds, drugs and xenobiotics, and consequently result in an individual's susceptibility to cancer.[136] In another study, Sulfotransferase 1A1 was up-regulated in plasma of hypobaric hypoxia treated rats. Other proteins detected include nucleoside diphosphate kinase (NME), a multifunctional enzyme involved in the maintenance of the cellular pools of nucleoside triphosphate and in transcriptional regulation.[137] Nucleoside diphosphate kinase has been shown to undergo S-thiolation or disulfide cross-linking under conditions of oxidative stress, which could have implications in function switching.[138] In this study, NME was up-regulated, suggesting the protective role against the oxidative stress induced by hypobaric hypoxia. In this experiment, candidate proteins corresponding to spots 6, 7 and 27 could not be detected in the database. They may be novel proteins, or else they may be small fragments of some proteins, as can be suggested from their low molecular weight. The ESI-MS/MS study of these spots may lead us to identify these novel proteins. Readers are advised to read the detailed study[139] at http://journals.plos.org/plosone/article?id=10.1371/journal.pone.0098027.

4.3   Human Plasma Proteome and Adaptation to High Altitudes

Man exposed to high altitude hypoxia is a convenient model for investigations on hypoxia mediated molecular changes particularly the proteome analysis. The advantage of a proteomic rather than a transcriptomic approach is that protein expression levels are measured directly, rather than being inferred from abundance of the corresponding mRNAs, which are imperfectly correlated to protein concentration[140] because of variable rates of synthesis and differences in message stability[141]. In fact, it allows identifying among several thousand proteins in plasma the molecular players undergoing significant changes as a function of a set of important variables of physiological interest (such as duration and degree of hypoxia, acid–base imbalance, nutritional habits, training, and exercise levels) known to influence the profiles of general and local oxygen partial pressure. Next after studying plasma proteome of rat we focused on, the changes in plasma proteome of human especially among high altitude natives and healthy control individuals were compared by 2-DE and MS. The results showed that most of the plasma proteins found in high altitude natives are acute phase proteins (APPs), compliment components and apolipoprotein and so on. These molecular variables may play important roles in the adpative process that could be of paramount importance to shed light on the mechanisms known to counteract the negative effects of oxygen lack.

The expression levels of 35 protein spots, which were identified by MALDI-TOF/TOF, showed significant changes in high altitude natives compared with controls. Several identified proteins related to oxidative and cellular defense mechanisms involving anti-inflammatory and antioxidant activity were the most common. The identified biological/cellular functions represent relevant targets for the adaptation processes under the influence of hypobaric hypox Vitamin D-binding protein (VDBP) belongs to the albumin superfamily of binding proteins that includes albumin, a-albumin, and a-fetoprotein. In addition, VDBP also mediates inflammatory and immunoregulatory activities in response to environmental challenges. Given the diverse and physiologically important roles of VDBP, down-regulation could contribute to a variety of health concerns.[142] Reduced levels of DBP have been observed in trauma patients who go on to develop organ dysfunction and sepsis, with complete depletion of free DBP in septic shock and hepatic necrosis being associated with a fatal outcome.[143] In this study, the high level of VDBP in high altitude natives may reflect its role as a scavenger protein or of protection against inflammation and might contribute to the mechanism of adaptation at high altitude hypoxia.

Hemoproteins undergo degradation during hypoxic/ischemic conditions, but the pro-oxidant free heme that is released cannot be recycled and must be degraded. The extracellular heme associates with its high-affinity binding protein, hemopexin (HPX). Hemopexin is the important constituent of iron homeostasis system, regulating cellular iron levels. It is mainly expressed in liver, and belongs to acute phase reactants, the synthesis of which is induced after inflammation. Heme is potentially highly toxic because of its ability to intercalate into lipid membrane and to produce hydroxyl radicals. The binding strength between heme and HPX, and the presence of a specific heme-HPX receptor able to catabolize the complex and to induce intracellular antioxidant activities, suggest that hemopexin is the major vehicle for the transportation of heme in the plasma, thus preventing heme-mediated oxidative stress and heme-bound iron loss.

A previous study has reported that genetic deletion of HPX significantly increases the severity of the brain damage from ischemic stroke, that heme–HPX protects cells and particularly neurons against both heme- and oxidative stress-induced toxicity.[144] In this study, we found that the plasma concentration of HPX was increased significantly, suggesting the most important physiological role as an antioxidant in high altitude natives by maintaining the tight balance between free and bound heme. A further interesting protein identified in high altitude natives was alpha-1-antitrypsin (SERPINA 1). It plays an important role in wound-healing, inhibiting plasmin and activating plasminogen and thrombin, and also inhibits hematopoietic stem cell mobilization in bone marrow. Further, in vitro studies showed an increase of lipopolysaccharide-mediated macrophage activation and anti-inflammatory effects on B-cells, demonstrating an additional role in immune regulation.[145] Major functions of the protein are to inactivate neutrophil elastase and other proteases to maintain a protease-antiprotease balance[146] to protect connective tissue of the lung from degradation by elastase, and to prevent the destruction of pulmonary extracellular matrix. It was reported that progression of pulmonary hypertension was associated with increased serine elastase activity.

Another protein whose expression was different in plasma from high altitude natives compared with that from sea level controls was haptoglobin. Haptoglobin (HP) is an acute phase reactant protein that functions as an antioxidant by virtue of its ability to bind to haemoglobin[147] and thereby to prevent the oxidative tissue damage that may be mediated by free haemoglobin[148]. The importance of this protective mechanism has been demonstrated in haptoglobin knockout mice in which a marked increase in oxidative tissue damage develops in response to hemolysis[147].

Haptoglobin consists of two different polypeptide chains: a and b chains.[149] The b chain (40 kDa) is heavier than the a chain and is identical in all the Hp types.[150] In our study we detected nine haptoglobin spots with an apparent experimental mass of 45 kDa, which suggests the presence of the haptoglobin b chain. The expression level of haptoglobin b is regulated by several cytokines, including IL-1, IL-6, TNF-a, and TGF-b. Plasma expression of haptoglobin b chain was significantly increased in high altitude natives compared with that from healthy sea level controls, suggesting the protective role as an antioxidant against the oxidative damage caused by hypobaric hypoxia.

Apolipoprotein A-I (APOA1, spot no: 19–21 and 31–33) was also identified in high altitude natives by comparison with controls. It belongs to the APOA1/A4/E protein family and is primarily produced in the liver and the intestine. APOA1 can be found in the extracellular space and, being a structural component of high density lipoprotein (HDL), takes part in cholesterol absorption. APOA1 up-regulation is associated with breast and lung cancer as suggested elsewhere.[151] APOA1 is also linked to antioxidant function that is proposed to be involved in its vasculo-protective activity, apparently by complexing with paraoxonase.[152] Interestingly, studies provide new evidence supporting the notion that HDL plays a protective role in the lung. ABCA1, which interacts with lipid-poor APOA1, was earlier shown to be essential for maintaining normal lipid composition and architecture of the lung as well as respiratory physiology.[153] There is emerging evidence that, APOA1 plays a critical role in protecting pulmonary artery and airway function as well as preventing inflammation and collagen deposition in the lung[37]. More recently, proteomic studies revealed the anti-inflammatory role of APOA1 in HAPE patients.[154] Here we report APOA1expression was up-regulated in high altitude natives suggesting the antiinflammatory role of APOA1.

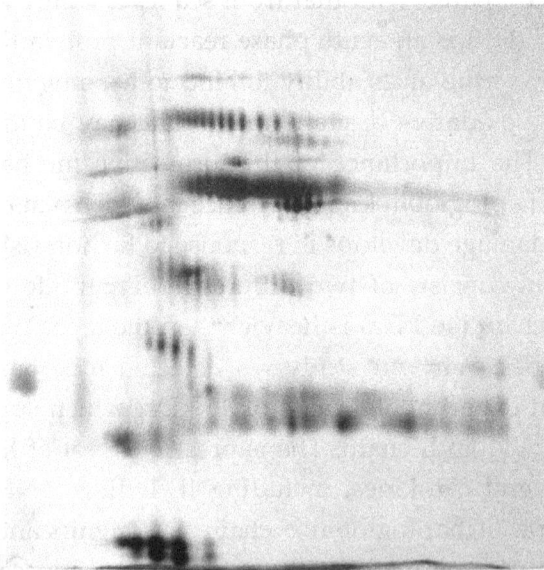

Figure 4.2: representative 2D gel electrophoresis gel stained using silver staining.

In summary, proteomic analysis of plasma from high altitude natives allowed the confident identification of several differentially expressed proteins in comparison to normal plasma. The proteomic information derived from the proteins detected in an increased or decreased level to determine if their protein expression signature could predict an adaptive response to hypobaric hypoxia in the plasma of high altitude natives. Interpreting the biological significance of these differences in protein expression is not an easy task but according to literature and current findings these proteins had a relatively high abundance in the plasma, and they all play a positive antiinflammatory role. The results show that there is some adaptive mechanism that sustains the inflammation balance and the homeostasis of the body in high altitude natives, thereby facilitating physical activity under extreme conditions. Importantly, we report 35 proteins with altered proteomic patterns in the plasma of high altitude natives, opening the door to further identification of mechanisms involved in hypobaric hypoxia and to their potential assessment as novel protein markers. Readers are advised to read the complete study[154] at http://link.springer.com/article/10.1007%2Fs10142-011-0234-3.

4.4   Perturbations in Rat Lung Proteome during Hypoxia Exposure

The lung is a unique tissue compared with many other vital organs since it is directly exposed to high levels of oxygen. One of the most important functions of lungs is to maintain an adequate oxygenation in the organism. This organ can be affected by hypoxia facing both physiological and pathological situations. Exposure to hypoxia results in the increase of reactive oxygen species from mitochondria, as from NADPH oxidase, xanthine oxidase/reductase, and nitric oxide synthase enzymes, as well as establishing an inflammatory process. In lungs, hypoxia also alters the levels of antioxidant substances causing pulmonary oxidative damage. Imbalance of redox state in lungs induced by hypoxia has been suggested as one of the causal factors for the changes in lung function in the hypoxic context, such as hypoxic vasoconstriction[155] and pulmonary edema[156] in addition to vascular remodeling and chronic pulmonary hypertension[58] Recently, discovery proteomics has emerged as a means of qualitatively differentiating specific proteins within complex samples such as lung or lung lavage fluid.

Compared to microarray based analysis of gene expression patterns, which has already been undertaken in hypoxic lung[157], proteomic profiling offers distinct advantages. When applied to hypoxic lung, discovery proteomics not only has the potential to provide insight into the key effectors of lung inflammation/injury and repair, but also uncover mechanisms regulating gene expression. Research involving proteomics methods have been applied to the study of hypoxic lung by several groups of investigators. Henschke and co-workers used an electrophoresis-based proteomic method to elucidate the effects of hyperoxia on protein expression in fetal rabbit lungs and to identify putative response pathways that mediates antioxidant and inflammatory processes.[158] Laudi and colleagues compared the *in vivo* changes in the lung proteome in monocrotaline and hypoxia induced pulmonary hypertension using 2-DE coupled with nanoflow LC-MS/MS to study the differences in the underlying mechanism of the regulation of vasoconstriction and remodeling.[159] Kwapiszewska and co-workers used a shotgun proteomic approach to identify chloride intracellular channel 4, as a novel multifunctional protein involved in angiogenesis and several signalling pathways implicated in pulmonary arterial hypertension.[160] Recently, lung proteome profiles of chronic hypoxic rats with pulmonary hypertension were compared with normoxic rats using 2D-based proteomics approach to identify the novel signalling pathways involved in the pathophysiology of pulmonary hypertension.[161]

Most recently, Olmeda *et al.* reported a proteomic approach to describe the changes in protein complement induced by moderate long-term hypoxia (rats exposed to 10% O2 for 72 h) in BAL and lung tissue, with a special focus on the protein associated with pulmonary surfactant[162]. These studies applied proteomics techniques to study proteins in lung exposed only to chronic hypoxia at a single time point but they did not address the complex and dynamic changes that occur during the course of hypoxia at different time points. Thus, the purpose of this study was to use proteomic analysis to profile the proteomic changes in the lungs exposed to short-term temporal (0, 6, 12 and 24 h) hypobaric hypoxia and hence, to identify the pathways that are affected due to hypoxia induced lung inflammation. We used a 2D- based proteomic approach to compare the protein profiles in the lung of rat treated with hypobaric hypoxia at different exposure time points. Several hypoxia-regulated proteins were identified by MALDI TOF/TOF. We then applied advanced methods in computational analysis to map complex protein interactions in the lung exposed to hypobaric hypoxia and studied how these interactions changed during the different exposure time points. This approach to protein network analysis identified novel mediators of acute lung hypoxia which were involved in multiple biological processes. These characteristics of the protein interactions in the lungs of rats treated with hypobaric hypoxia have important implications for the development of new molecular-based therapies.

5

Future Guidelines

Given the scale and challenges of hypobaric hypoxia (as described in chapter 2) have reported specific changes in physiological parameters including fluid leakage, memory/cognition that can be distinctively observed by 18–24 h of hypobaric hypoxia exposure. Since the final outcome of the high altitude exposure majorly depends on the duration of stay, it is important to decipher the temporal proteomic changes in lung tissue for better understanding of sequential cascade of molecular events regulated by hypobaric hypoxia. Moreover, comparison of proteome profiles will provide a molecular insight into differential hypoxia response of lung proteins in rats. Those studies reveal, for the first time, major alterations in expression level of newly identified proteins, regucalcin, sulfotransferase 1A1, Keratin, type I cytoskeletal 10 and other proteins. The identified proteins in hypoxic lung are involved in specific biological processes (inflammation, immunity, oxidative stress, haemostasis and signalling) and potentially implicated in the pathogenesis of hypoxia induced lung injury/inflammation. The confirmation of these specific protein in the plasma of HAPE patients and healthy control subjects has demonstrated their discrimatory power of HAPE detection. Although further validation in a larger sample set is necessary for biomarker discovery. Additionally, such discoveries promote new directions of thought and research regarding the pathophysiology of high altitude hypoxia related lung disease like HAPE, pathogenesis of complications involved in it, potential treatments targeting these proteomically identified aberrations, and earlier, and more specific, screening and diagnostic modalities. Future investigation in this area over the next five years holds promise for devising new biomarkers to predict prognosis of lung disease, stratify risk and provide surrogate outcome markers for future clinical trials in lung disease related to hypobaric hypoxia. Such biomarkers could help to guide risky curative therapies and also to accelerate drug development to reduce the burden of human suffering from high altitude illness. Readers are advised to read detailed study[163] at http://www.nature.com/articles/srep10681.

Despite of the major achievements as discussed in the preceding sections, there is still a gap between clinical conclusions and basic molecular research on hypobaric hypoxia. Most of the studies pertaining to the determination of biomarker for high altitude associated pathophysiology still remain to be validated at the larger sub-clinical and clinical scale. Although, therapeutic interventions for amelioration of disorders such as High altitude pulmonary edema (HAPE) or High altitude cerebral edema (HACE) have been established much before the current molecular biology research begun, however, the prophylactic strategies to prevent the occurrence of such event is still a challenge. If one begin to understand the reason behind partial success in prophylactic strategies, the poor understanding of the susceptibility is one common root cause. Previous genomic studies and proteomics studies have emerged as unclear answers to this questions by associating common genetic variations such as singe nucleotide polymorphism and copy number variations as possible answers to the question of susceptibility. If we look at the proteomic side of the answer then it is still very blurred and no significant work has been done on understanding the dynamics of protein function at reduced partial pressure of oxygen. On one hand where we now know that expression levels of many antioxidant and associated proteins are altered, we are unclear about the functional efficacies of proteins, which indicated the future scope of this domain. Similarly, on the clinical ground the detailed case studies of high altitude sickness are not poorly recorded and such data are not available to the global community. Therefore adding knowledge to this domain and using modern computational biology and machine learning algorithms we may achieve much better and higher goals in the high altitude biology. Below is the description of both these strategies in detail.

5.1   Answering Hypoxia Susceptibility: Computer Simulations

Structure- functional relationship of proteins is well known from the more than five decades. Many of the in silico programs are now available that may help in understanding the dynamics of proteins under varying solvent conditions or during Biomolecular interactions. These studies work on the basic principles of calculating the force-field and interaction energies under various conditions. Some of the common programs that are used for the study of molecular dynamics are listed below.

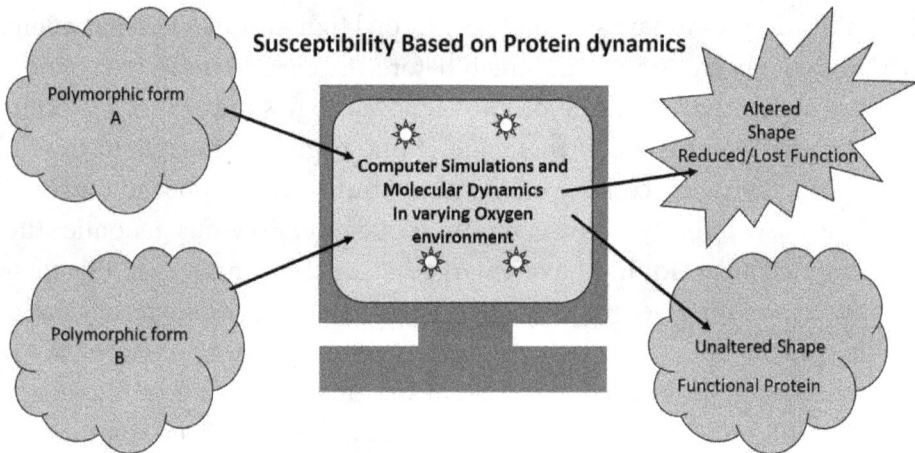

Figure 5.1: Molecular dynamic simulations using varying oxygen concentrations in silico may be used to obtain a closed look at protein functioning during hypoxic environments.

Many proteins especially those circulating in the blood are affected by the saturation of oxygen. Hemoglobin is well studied protein that differs in its conformations at varying oxygen saturation and shows a charactertic saturation kinetics. But many other proteins which do not directly interact with the oxygen may also be affected by the saturation of oxygen in the blood by some indirect means. The altered levels of oxygen in the high altitude stimulate the compensatory cardiovascular response, which result in the hyperventilation (more number of breath per unit time to compensate low oxygen saturation). This results in the decreased reduced partial pressure of carbon di oxide which is a major buffering system in the blood and eventually ends up in slight decrease in the pH of blood, commonly called as **respiratory alkalosis**. As the ionization state of the amino acids is largely dependent on the pH of surrounding, it is speculated that such events are likely to occur during compensatory responses. These changes may be reflected at a larger level in the form of conformational changes in the proteins.

Another critical factors that is known from the polymorphism studies indicates that small changes/substitutions in the amino acids occurring due to single nucleotide polymorphism may also results in the altered geometry of protein at active site or regulatory site and therefore may directly influence the efficacy of that protein . Such studies have not been done yet and if assisted with newer computer simulations that consider oxygen saturation in force filed calculations could be a value addition to the current proteomics conformation gathered on high altitude pathophysiology.

5.2   Machine Learning, Cloud Computing and AI for Developing Improved Scoring for Altitude Sickness

Plethora of scientific information is now available on diagnosis and therapy of HAPE and if detected on time it is curable, yet we do not have a precise answer for HAPE susceptibility. Involvement of genetic, epigenetic, physiological and other associated factors in deciding the HAPE susceptibility poses a major challenge for the scientific resolution of the problem. With the advancement and accessibility to high throughput omics technologies, genome-wide data sets and description of susceptibility architecture, translational research in high altitude medicine will be an important aspect of medical progress. Global metabolite profiling combined with a systems biology approach (i.e., integrating genomics, epigenomics, and proteomics) is an exciting upcoming approach for improving our understanding of HAPE and evaluating various potential biomarkers for the same. As a futuristic vision, developments in modelling of computer simulations of various biological networks to investigate "what if" questions about real world systems may provide implantable solution for susceptibility assessment. Furthermore, this could be extended to cloud based screening of aforesaid biomarkers and development of HAPE susceptibility scoring based on the machine learning or artificial intelligence[164]. Now let us understand few aspects of machine learning and then we will discuss the future possibilities of using it in high altitude research.

Machine learning is a computer assisted method which helps machine to analyse and curate a data set based on previous task history. Machine learning can be of two types supervised and unsupervised as described below. Additionally newer methods that are used for machine learning include artificial neural network (ANN) and support vector machines (SVM).

Unsupervised approaches are simplest routine approach to visualize the distribution of data. These approaches include k-means clustering, principal component analysis (PCA), and hierarchical clustering which can be used a basis for feature selection. PCA maps high dimensional data by creating eigenvalues. Each linear combination or principal component is a weighted sum of the amplitude at each m/z value. The feature selections of PCA are present in the top principal components which separates the samples into homogeneous clusters and can be visualized in 2D or in 3D plots in which the calculated values for top principal components serve as x, y, and z axes. The PCA approach was used to rank peak intensities within each spectrum and applied on cervical [165] and borderline ovarian cancers [166]. Hierarchical clustering (HC) is another powerful data mining method for initial exploration of proteomic data. HC begins by assigning each sample to its own cluster. It further calculates similarity scores or distance matrices between sample and places samples that are close to each other. HC algorithms may differ in calculating distance matrices. Two way clustering algorithm was used to differentiate cancerous from non-cancerous cells and human CSF[167-169].

Supervised learning techniques require class labels such that training can occur on data obtained from a subset of the provided samples. The two types of variables in this exercise are predictor variables (intensity at m/z values or peak intensity) and a response variable (disease). The straight approach to identify the difference between two groups would be a t-test using a supervised method. Unlike Welch t-test, Mann-Whitney test assumes equal variance between the two groups. The t-test has some limitations like by calculating t-statistics for each peak, multiple testing can give more number of variables, and these calculations assume that measurements are independent of each other. Bonferroni correction reduces the impact of multiple testing procedure.[170] Classification algorithms can be used for feature selection and classification. Such algorithms include genetic algorithms, decision trees, and neural networks. The aim of genetic algorithms (GA) is to extract a model by creating chromosomes of input variables (m/z values) and iteratively recombining chromosomes and mutating genes. More specifically, this mathematical model relates the protein abundance with the presence of a certain gene. This process progressively becomes more difficult as the number of variables grow. Input variables that satisfy fitness function are kept and the rest are discarded through computational evolution. GA have been used in various MS datasets [171]. Petricoin et.al used GA and self-organizing maps (SOM) and applied these to the development of diagnostic patterns for ovarian and prostate cancers to find a good set of predictive SELDI *m/z* values[172].

Artifical neural networks are based on the way the human brain processes information. Neurons integerate information obtained from different inputs which could be outside world (primary level data) or previously integrated data (other neurons). Most neural networks feed forward, i.e., information flow is unidirectional, starting with an input layer flowing through n layer of neurons and finally to the output. Training the neural network involves decreasing the error rate by adjusting model parameters, i.e., assigning weights to input function, activation threshold of each neuron, and computation function performed by each neuron. Due to their low error rates, artificial neural network algorithms have been applied to analyze mass spectra for cancer and neurodegenerative diseases [167,173].

Support Vector machines is another machine learning approach which is applied to MS data analysis. SVMs operate first by distributing the sample in n-dimensional space and then by finding a hyperspace that attempts to split the cases from controls samples. Numerous studies have used SVMs for MS data analysis[117,174,175].

A simple strategy could be used to enhance the previous scoring systems and the susceptibility could be redefined in better terms. A global network of clinicians encountering high altitude patients, agencies handing high altitude travelers and clinicians at high altitude hospitals may be integrated through a network of computers and a common database accepting the inputs about the physiological parameters of healthy and unhealthy individuals may be added to the database on recurring basis. This information will then be processed and analysed by cloud based machine learning and Artificial intelligence protocol and new conclusions like de-

pendence of a particular SNP with susceptibility, presence of specific pro-
tein/metabolite in blood as an indicator of susceptibility will be known.
Figure 5.2 depicts the outline of cloud based computing and AI for development of newer scoring systems for high altitude sickness.

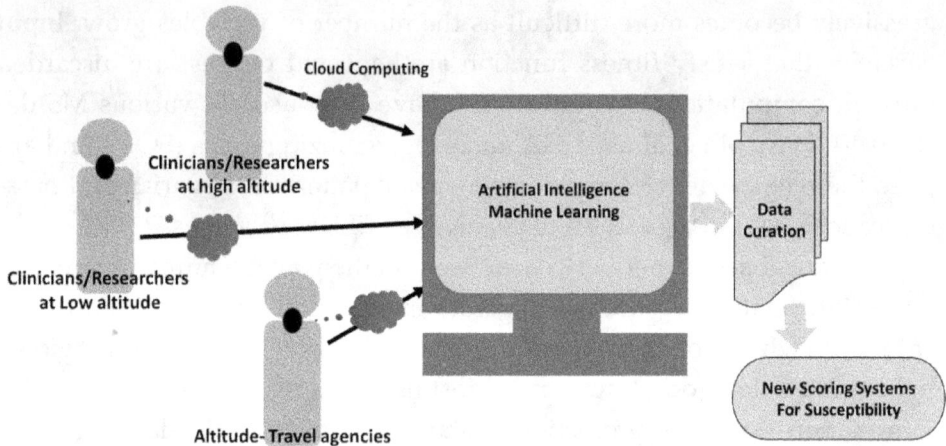

Figure 5.2: Cloud based clinical data accumulation and its analysis by machine learning and artificial intelligence can support the faster discovery of
novel biomarkers and aid in developing new scoring systems.

Readers must note that significantly reliable cure and therapeutic interventions are available for high altitude associated disorders and even a
rapid decent to lower altitude benefits the patients, but the bigger question
that need to answered is the susceptibility and development of prophylactic strategies. Which should be prime focus of the high altitude-
pathophysiology.

5.3   Novel Biosensors for Determination of Susceptibility

Biosensors are defined as devices that are made up of a transducer and a
biological component (enzyme, antibody or nucleic acid) and helps in detection a metabolite (qualitative and quantitative). A biosensor consist of
three major components: a **bioreceptor**, a **tranducer** and a **signal pro-**

cessing system. Biosensors may be classified on the basis of type of bioreceptor or type of transducer.

Bioreceptors is a molecule that utilizes a biological mechanism for recognition. They assist in the binding of analyte of interest to the sensor surface for the measurement. Commonly used Bioreceptors include enzymes, antibody/antigen, nucleic acid/DNA, cellular structures and a biomimetic. The sampling component of a biosensor contains a bio-sensitive layer that contains bioreceptor or be made of bioreceptor covalently attached to the transducer. The enzymes and the antibodies are the most widely used form of Bioreceptors. Transducer is second component of the biosensor that plays and important role in the signal transduction process. It converts bio-recognition signal event into detectable signals. The detectable signals can be electrochemical (potentiometric, conductometric, amperometric or voltametric), optical (colorimetric, flurimetric, luminometric), calorimetric, piezoelectric or magnetic in nature. A signal processing system is primarily made of an analog to digital converter that processes analog data acquired from a transducer and thus making it available to the user in the digital form that may be further used to compare with standards and quantitate the data.

Under hypoxic environment especially hypobaric hypoxia, previous proteomics studies have indicated a large number of proteins being altered in terms of their concentrations. This information can be directly used to correlate and perform the diagnosis of high altitude illness. Similarly, baseline difference some of the proteins also hint at the varying trend in the susceptibility of individuals towards high altitude sickness and thus could be used to predict the same. Biosensors could be a quantum leap in the area of hypobaric –hypoxia research and thefore more thrust should be given for the development of portable and cost effective biosensors. The design and development of biosensors may be based on the simple principles of signal transduction and integrating with the information arising from basing proteomic or genomic research. At this point of time when enough confidence has not yet been achieved in biomarker for High altitude sickness diagnosis and susceptibility, biosensor design may be useful for validation of putative biomarkers on the larger scales. Two basic strategies may be used to develop biosensors, one based on the proteomic information emerging from the comparison of healthy individuals and patients of high altitude sickness which will be useful for diagnostic purpose.

The other set of biosensors may be prepared for the evaluation of susceptibility of high altitude sickness. In such biosensors the information emerging from the genomic or proteomic studies that are performed on high altitude native, low land mountain travelers may be used.

A newer mode of biosensors called lab-on-a chip is also emerging and in such kind of biosensors multiple biomolecules may be assessed. However, this strategy is still much advanced and need much more proteomic and metabolomic information form high altitude studies especially on the dynamics of proteins such as temporal and spatial variation in protein levels and the kinetic parameters of the metabolites during aforesaid environmental conditions.

Following figure (Figure 5.3) depicts the scheme of biosensor development and how it will benefit the hypobaric- hypoxia research.

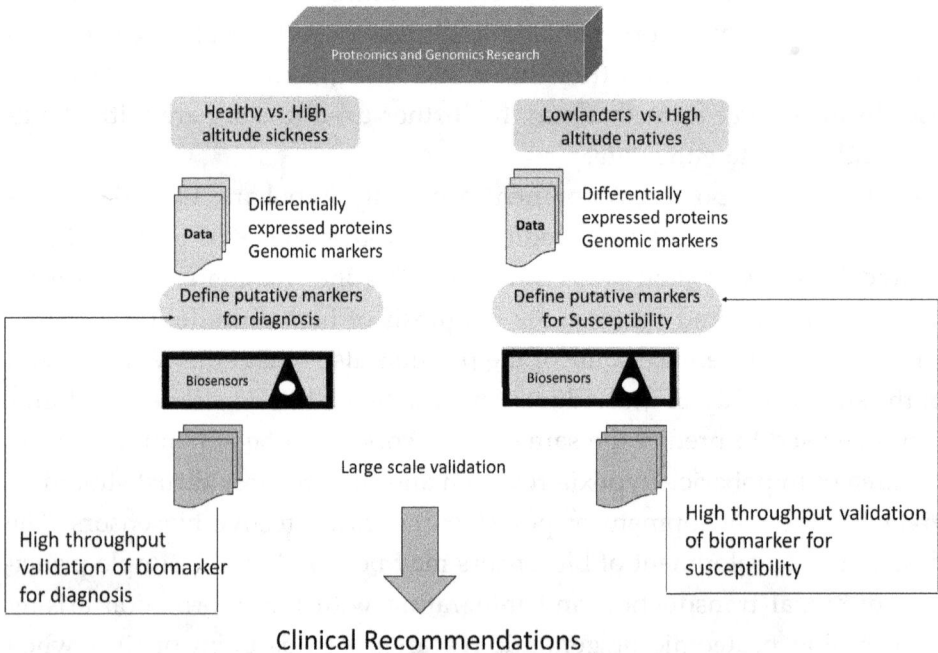

Figure 5.3: Design and development of biosensors based on the information accumulated from genomics and proteomics studies on high altitude

Acknowledgement

Aditya Arya would like to acknowledge Council of Scientific and Industrial Research (CSIR), New Delhi, India for Senior Research Fellowship. The Photographs of MALDI-TOF, isoelectric focusing unit and 2D gel were kindly provided by **Ms. Shikha Jain,** Junior Research Fellow, Peptide and Proteomics Lab, DIPAS, DRDO, Delhi. Image of the coomasie stained 1D gel was kindly provide by **Ms. Anamika Gangwar,** DST-INSPIRE-Senior Research Fellow, Peptide and Proteomics Lab, DIPAS, DRDO, Delhi.

References

1   Bakonyi, T. & Radak, Z. High altitude and free radicals. *J Sports Sci Med* **3**, 64-69 (2004).

2   Teppema, L. J. & Dahan, A. The ventilatory response to hypoxia in mammals: mechanisms, measurement, and analysis. *Physiological reviews* **90**, 675-754, doi:10.1152/physrev.00012.2009 (2010).

3   Hackett, P. H. & Roach, R. C. High altitude cerebral edema. *High altitude medicine & biology* **5**, 136-146, doi:10.1089/1527029041352054 (2004).

4   Wilson, M. H., Newman, S. & Imray, C. H. The cerebral effects of ascent to high altitudes. *Lancet Neurol* **8**, 175-191, doi:10.1016/S1474-4422(09)70014-6 (2009).

5   West, J. B. T.H. Ravenhill and his contributions to mountain sickness. *J Appl Physiol (1985)* **80**, 715-724 (1996).

6   Hackett, P. H., Roach, R. C., Hartig, G. S., Greene, E. R. & Levine, B. D. The effect of vasodilators on pulmonary hemodynamics in high altitude pulmonary edema: a comparison. *Int J Sports Med* **13 Suppl 1**, S68-71, doi:10.1055/s-2007-1024599 (1992).

7   Marticorena, E. & Hultgren, H. N. Evaluation of therapeutic methods in high altitude pulmonary edema. *Am J Cardiol* **43**, 307-312 (1979).

8   Vock, P., Brutsche, M. H., Nanzer, A. & Bartsch, P. Variable radio-morphologic data of high altitude pulmonary edema. Features from 60 patients. *Chest* **100**, 1306-1311 (1991).

9   Hultgren, H. N. High-altitude pulmonary edema: current concepts. *Annu Rev Med* **47**, 267-284, doi:10.1146/annurev.med.47.1.267 (1996).

10   Penaloza, D. & Sime, F. Circulatory dynamics during high altitude pulmonary edema. *Am J Cardiol* **23**, 369-378 (1969).

11   Allemann, Y. *et al.* Echocardiographic and invasive measurements of pulmonary artery pressure correlate closely at high altitude. *Am J Physiol Heart Circ Physiol* **279**, H2013-2016 (2000).

12   Zhao, L. *et al.* Sildenafil inhibits hypoxia-induced pulmonary hypertension. *Circulation* **104**, 424-428 (2001).

13   Maggiorini, M. *et al.* High-altitude pulmonary edema is initially caused by an increase in capillary pressure. *Circulation* **103**, 2078-2083 (2001).

14   Schoene, R. B. *et al.* The lung at high altitude: bronchoalveolar lavage in acute mountain sickness and pulmonary edema. *J Appl Physiol (1985)* **64**, 2605-2613 (1988).

15   Swenson, E. R. & Maggiorini, M. Salmeterol for the prevention of high-altitude pulmonary edema. *The New England journal of medicine* **347**, 1282-1285; author reply 1282-1285 (2002).

16   Sutton, J. R. Mountain sickness. *Neurol Clin* **10**, 1015-1030 (1992).

17   Yarnell, P. R., Heit, J. & Hackett, P. H. High-altitude cerebral edema (HACE): the Denver/Front Range experience. *Semin Neurol* **20**, 209-217, doi:10.1055/s-2000-9830 (2000).

18   Hackett, P. H., Roach, R. C., Schoene, R. B., Harrison, G. L. & Mills, W. J., Jr. Abnormal control of ventilation in high-altitude pulmonary edema. *J Appl Physiol (1985)* **64**, 1268-1272 (1988).

19   Savonitto, S. *et al.* Effects of acute exposure to altitude (3,460 m) on blood pressure response to dynamic and isometric exercise in men with systemic hypertension. *Am J Cardiol* **70**, 1493-1497 (1992).

20   Wu, T. Y. *et al.* High-altitude gastrointestinal bleeding: an observation in Qinghai-Tibetan railroad construction workers on Mountain Tanggula. *World J Gastroenterol* **13**, 774-780 (2007).

21   Chandel, N. S. *et al.* Mitochondrial reactive oxygen species trigger hypoxia-induced transcription. *Proceedings of the National Academy of Sciences of the United States of America* **95**, 11715-11720 (1998).

22   Chandel, N. S. *et al.* Reactive oxygen species generated at mito-chondrial complex III stabilize hypoxia-inducible factor-1alpha during hypoxia: a mechanism of O2 sensing. *The Journal of biological chemistry* **275**, 25130-25138, doi:10.1074/jbc.M001914200 (2000).

23   Guzy, R. D. *et al.* Mitochondrial complex III is required for hypoxia-induced ROS production and cellular oxygen sensing. *Cell metabolism* **1**, 401-408, doi:10.1016/j.cmet.2005.05.001 (2005).

24   Vaux, E. C., Metzen, E., Yeates, K. M. & Ratcliffe, P. J. Regulation of hypoxia-inducible factor is preserved in the absence of a functioning mitochondrial respiratory chain. *Blood* **98**, 296-302 (2001).

25   Srinivas, V. *et al.* Oxygen sensing and HIF-1 activation does not require an active mitochondrial respiratory chain electron-transfer pathway. *The Journal of biological chemistry* **276**, 21995-21998, doi:10.1074/jbc.C100177200 (2001).

26   Bell, E. L. & Chandel, N. S. Mitochondrial oxygen sensing: regulation of hypoxia-inducible factor by mitochondrial generated reactive oxygen species. *Essays in biochemistry* **43**, 17-27, doi:10.1042/BSE0430017 (2007).

27   Bell, E. L., Klimova, T. A., Eisenbart, J., Schumacker, P. T. & Chandel, N. S. Mitochondrial reactive oxygen species trigger hypoxia-inducible factor-dependent extension of the replicative life span during hypoxia. *Molecular and cellular biology* **27**, 5737-5745, doi:10.1128/MCB.02265-06 (2007).

28   Na, N., Chandel, N. S., Litvan, J. & Ridge, K. M. Mitochondrial reactive oxygen species are required for hypoxia-induced degradation of keratin intermediate filaments. *FASEB journal: official publication of the Federation of American Societies for Experimental Biology* **24**, 799-809, doi:10.1096/fj.08-128967 (2010).

29   Smith, T. G., Robbins, P. A. & Ratcliffe, P. J. The human side of hypoxia-inducible factor. *British journal of haematology* **141**, 325-334, doi:10.1111/j.1365-2141.2008.07029.x (2008).

30   Jiang, B. H., Semenza, G. L., Bauer, C. & Marti, H. H. Hypoxia-inducible factor 1 levels vary exponentially over a physiologically relevant range of O2 tension. *The American journal of physiology* **271**, C1172-1180 (1996).

31   Greer, S. N., Metcalf, J. L., Wang, Y. & Ohh, M. The updated biology of hypoxia-inducible factor. *The EMBO journal* **31**, 2448-2460, doi:10.1038/emboj.2012.125 (2012).

32   Semenza, G. L. *et al.* Hypoxia response elements in the aldolase A, enolase 1, and lactate dehydrogenase A gene promoters contain essential binding sites for hypoxia-inducible factor 1. *The Journal of biological chemistry* **271**, 32529-32537 (1996).

33   Majmundar, A. J., Wong, W. J. & Simon, M. C. Hypoxia-inducible factors and the response to hypoxic stress. *Molecular cell* **40**, 294-309, doi:10.1016/j.molcel.2010.09.022 (2010).

34   Stroka, D. M. *et al.* HIF-1 is expressed in normoxic tissue and displays an organ-specific regulation under systemic hypoxia. *FASEB journal: official publication of the Federation of American Societies for Experimental Biology* **15**, 2445-2453, doi:10.1096/fj.01-0125com (2001).

35   Elbarghati, L., Murdoch, C. & Lewis, C. E. Effects of hypoxia on transcription factor expression in human monocytes and macrophages. *Immunobiology* **213**, 899-908, doi:10.1016/j.imbio.2008.07.016 (2008).

36   Fangradt, M. *et al.* Human monocytes and macrophages differ in their mechanisms of adaptation to hypoxia. *Arthritis research & therapy* **14**, R181, doi:10.1186/ar4011 (2012).

37   Wang, G. L. & Semenza, G. L. Purification and characterization of hypoxia-inducible factor 1. *The Journal of biological chemistry* **270**, 1230-1237 (1995).

38   Peng, Y. J. *et al.* Heterozygous HIF-1alpha deficiency impairs carotid body-mediated systemic responses and reactive oxygen species generation in mice exposed to intermittent hypoxia. *The Journal of physiology* **577**, 705-716, doi:10.1113/jphysiol.2006.114033 (2006).

39   Vaux, E. C. *et al.* Selection of mutant CHO cells with constitutive activation of the HIF system and inactivation of the von Hippel-Lindau tumor suppressor. *The Journal of biological chemistry* **276**, 44323-44330, doi:10.1074/jbc.M104678200 (2001).

40   Knowles, H. J., Mole, D. R., Ratcliffe, P. J. & Harris, A. L. Normoxic stabilization of hypoxia-inducible factor-1alpha by modulation of the labile iron pool in differentiating U937 macrophages: effect of natural resistance-associated macrophage protein 1. *Cancer research* **66**, 2600-2607, doi:10.1158/0008-5472.CAN-05-2351 (2006).

41   Ponti, A., Machacek, M., Gupton, S. L., Waterman-Storer, C. M. & Danuser, G. Two distinct actin networks drive the protrusion of migrating cells. *Science* **305**, 1782-1786, doi:10.1126/science.1100533 (2004).

42   Patten, D. A. *et al.* Hypoxia-inducible factor-1 activation in non-hypoxic conditions: the essential role of mitochondrial-derived reactive oxygen species. *Molecular biology of the cell* **21**, 3247-3257, doi:10.1091/mbc.E10-01-0025 (2010).

43   Atkuri, K. R., Herzenberg, L. A., Niemi, A. K. & Cowan, T. Importance of culturing primary lymphocytes at physiological oxygen levels. *Proceedings of the National Academy of Sciences of the United States of America* **104**, 4547-4552, doi:10.1073/pnas.0611732104 (2007).

44   Frede, S., Stockmann, C., Freitag, P. & Fandrey, J. Bacterial lipopolysaccharide induces HIF-1 activation in human monocytes via p44/42 MAPK and NF-kappaB. *The Biochemical journal* **396**, 517-527, doi:10.1042/BJ20051839 (2006).

45   Benizri, E., Ginouves, A. & Berra, E. The magic of the hypoxia-signaling cascade. *Cellular and molecular life sciences: CMLS* **65**, 1133-1149, doi:10.1007/s00018-008-7472-0 (2008).

46   Goda, N. *et al.* Hypoxia-inducible factor 1alpha is essential for cell cycle arrest during hypoxia. *Molecular and cellular biology* **23**, 359-369 (2003).

47   Koshiji, M. *et al.* HIF-1alpha induces cell cycle arrest by functionally counteracting Myc. *The EMBO journal* **23**, 1949-1956, doi:10.1038/sj.emboj.7600196 (2004).

48   Seoane, J., Le, H. V. & Massague, J. Myc suppression of the p21(Cip1) Cdk inhibitor influences the outcome of the p53 response to DNA damage. *Nature* **419**, 729-734, doi:10.1038/nature01119 (2002).

49   Herold, S. *et al.* Negative regulation of the mammalian UV response by Myc through association with Miz-1. *Molecular cell* **10**, 509-521 (2002).

50   Sclafani, R. A. & Holzen, T. M. Cell cycle regulation of DNA replication. *Annual review of genetics* **41**, 237-280, doi:10.1146/annurev.genet.41.110306.130308 (2007).

51   Hubbi, M. E., Luo, W., Baek, J. H. & Semenza, G. L. MCM proteins are negative regulators of hypoxia-inducible factor 1. *Molecular cell* **42**, 700-712, doi:10.1016/j.molcel.2011.03.029 (2011).

52   Kaelin, W. G., Jr. & Ratcliffe, P. J. Oxygen sensing by metazoans: the central role of the HIF hydroxylase pathway. *Molecular cell* **30**, 393-402, doi:10.1016/j.molcel.2008.04.009 (2008).

53   Badr, M. S. *et al.* Ventilatory response to induced auditory arousals during NREM sleep. *Sleep* **20**, 707-714 (1997).

54   Cheng, S. Y. *et al.* Suppression of glioblastoma angiogenicity and tumorigenicity by inhibition of endogenous expression of vascular endothelial growth factor. *Proceedings of the National Academy of Sciences of the United States of America* **93**, 8502-8507 (1996).

55   Santore, M. T., McClintock, D. S., Lee, V. Y., Budinger, G. R. & Chandel, N. S. Anoxia-induced apoptosis occurs through a mitochondria-dependent pathway in lung epithelial cells. *American journal of physiology. Lung cellular and molecular physiology* **282**, L727-734, doi:10.1152/ajplung.00281.2001 (2002).

56   Forstermann, U. Nitric oxide and oxidative stress in vascular disease. *Pflugers Archiv: European journal of physiology* **459**, 923-939, doi:10.1007/s00424-010-0808-2 (2010).

57   Mueller, C. F., Laude, K., McNally, J. S. & Harrison, D. G. ATVB in focus: redox mechanisms in blood vessels. *Arteriosclerosis, thrombosis, and vascular biology* **25**, 274-278, doi:10.1161/01.ATV.0000149143.04821.eb (2005).

58   Radak, Z. *et al.* Superoxide dismutase derivative reduces oxidative damage in skeletal muscle of rats during exhaustive exercise. *J Appl Physiol (1985)* **79**, 129-135 (1995).

59   Halliwell, B. Free radicals, antioxidants, and human disease: curiosity, cause, or consequence? *Lancet* **344**, 721-724 (1994).

60   Freitas, R. M., Vasconcelos, S. M., Souza, F. C., Viana, G. S. & Fonteles, M. M. Oxidative stress in the hippocampus after pilocarpine-induced status epilepticus in Wistar rats. *The FEBS journal* **272**, 1307-1312, doi:10.1111/j.1742-4658.2004.04537.x (2005).

61   Powers, S. K. & Jackson, M. J. Exercise-induced oxidative stress: cellular mechanisms and impact on muscle force production. *Physiological reviews* **88**, 1243-1276, doi:10.1152/physrev.00031.2007 (2008).

62   Martasek, P. *et al.* The C331A mutant of neuronal nitric-oxide synthase is defective in arginine binding. *The Journal of biological chemistry* **273**, 34799-34805 (1998).

63   Fukui, T. *et al.* p22phox mRNA expression and NADPH oxidase activity are increased in aortas from hypertensive rats. *Circulation research* **80**, 45-51 (1997).

64   Hink, U. *et al.* Mechanisms underlying endothelial dysfunction in diabetes mellitus. *Circulation research* **88**, E14-22 (2001).

65   Warnholtz, A. *et al.* Increased NADH-oxidase-mediated superoxide production in the early stages of atherosclerosis: evidence for involvement of the renin-angiotensin system. *Circulation* **99**, 2027-2033 (1999).

66   Sorescu, D. & Griendling, K. K. Reactive oxygen species, mito-chondria, and NAD(P)H oxidases in the development and progression of heart failure. *Congest Heart Fail* **8**, 132-140 (2002).

67   Dikalova, A. *et al.* Nox1 overexpression potentiates angiotensin II-induced hypertension and vascular smooth muscle hypertrophy in transgenic mice. *Circulation* **112**, 2668-2676, doi:10.1161/circulationaha.105.538934 (2005).

68   Muller, F. L., Liu, Y. & Van Remmen, H. Complex III releases superoxide to both sides of the inner mitochondrial membrane. *The Journal of biological chemistry* **279**, 49064-49073, doi:10.1074/jbc.M407715200 (2004).

69   Ramachandran, A. *et al.* Mitochondria, nitric oxide, and cardiovascular dysfunction. *Free radical biology & medicine* **33**, 1465-1474 (2002).

70   Ballinger, S. W. Mitochondrial dysfunction in cardiovascular disease. *Free radical biology & medicine* **38**, 1278-1295, doi:10.1016/j.freeradbiomed.2005.02.014 (2005).

71   Ohashi, K. *et al.* Adiponectin replenishment ameliorates obesity-related hypertension. *Hypertension* **47**, 1108-1116, doi:10.1161/01.HYP.0000222368.43759.a1 (2006).

72   Stuehr, D. J. Mammalian nitric oxide synthases. *Biochimica et biophysica acta* **1411**, 217-230 (1999).

73   Bailey, S. J. *et al.* Dietary nitrate supplementation enhances muscle contractile efficiency during knee-extensor exercise in humans. *J Appl Physiol (1985)* **109**, 135-148, doi:10.1152/japplphysiol.00046.2010 (2010).

74   Pritchard, J. K., Stephens, M., Rosenberg, N. A. & Donnelly, P. Association mapping in structured populations. *American journal of human genetics* **67**, 170-181, doi:10.1086/302959 (2000).

75   Cosentino, F. *et al.* Tetrahydrobiopterin alters superoxide and nitric oxide release in prehypertensive rats. *The Journal of clinical investigation* **101**, 1530-1537, doi:10.1172/JCI650 (1998).

76   Kerr, B. & Myers, P. Withdrawal syndrome following long-term administration of tamoxifen. *J Psychopharmacol* **13**, 419 (1999).

77   Mollnau, H. *et al.* Effects of angiotensin II infusion on the expression and function of NAD(P)H oxidase and components of nitric oxide/cGMP signaling. *Circulation research* **90**, E58-65 (2002).

78   Stroes, E. *et al.* Tetrahydrobiopterin restores endothelial function in hypercholesterolemia. *The Journal of clinical investigation* **99**, 41-46, doi:10.1172/JCI119131 (1997).

79   Heitzer, T. *et al.* Beneficial effects of alpha-lipoic acid and ascorbic acid on endothelium-dependent, nitric oxide-mediated vasodilation in diabetic patients: relation to parameters of oxidative stress. *Free radical biology & medicine* **31**, 53-61 (2001).

80   Higashi, Y. *et al.* Endothelial function and oxidative stress in renovascular hypertension. *The New England journal of medicine* **346**, 1954-1962, doi:10.1056/NEJMoa013591 (2002).

81   Nakanishi, K. *et al.* Effects of hypobaric hypoxia on antioxidant enzymes in rats. *The Journal of physiology* **489 (Pt 3)**, 869-876 (1995).

82   Maiti, P. *et al.* Hypobaric hypoxia induces oxidative stress in rat brain. *Neurochem Int* **49**, 709-716, doi:10.1016/j.neuint.2006.06.002 (2006).

83   Arya, A., Sethy, N. K., Singh, S. K., Das, M. & Bhargava, K. Cerium oxide nanoparticles protect rodent lungs from hypobaric hypoxia-induced oxidative stress and inflammation. *Int J Nanomedicine* **8**, 4507-4520, doi:10.2147/IJN.S53032 (2013).

84   Singh, M., Arya, A., Kumar, R., Bhargava, K. & Sethy, N. K. Dietary nitrite attenuates oxidative stress and activates antioxidant genes in rat heart during hypobaric hypoxia. *Nitric Oxide* **26**, 61-73, doi: 10.1016/j.niox.2011.12.002 (2012).

85   Aviram, M. *et al.* Human serum paraoxonases (PON1) Q and R selectively decrease lipid peroxides in human coronary and carotid atherosclerotic lesions: PON1 esterase and peroxidase-like activities. *Circulation* **101**, 2510-2517 (2000).

86   Wilkins, M. R. & Williams, K. L. The extracellular matrix of the Dictyostelium discoideum slug. *Experientia* **51**, 1189-1196 (1995).

87   Lee, M. V. *et al.* A dynamic model of proteome changes reveals new roles for transcript alteration in yeast. *Molecular systems biology* **7**, 514, doi:10.1038/msb.2011.48 (2011).

88   Pagani, I. *et al.* The Genomes OnLine Database (GOLD) v.4: status of genomic and metagenomic projects and their associated metadata. *Nucleic acids research* **40**, D571-579, doi:10.1093/nar/gkr1100 (2012).

89   Devergne, J. C., Cardin, L., Burckard, J. & Van Regenmortel, M. H. Comparison of direct and indirect ELISA for detecting antigenically related cucumoviruses. *Journal of virological methods* **3**, 193-199 (1981).

90   Strimbu, K. & Tavel, J. A. What are biomarkers? *Current opinion in HIV and AIDS* **5**, 463-466, doi:10.1097/COH.0b013e32833ed177 (2010).

91   Group, B. D. W. Biomarkers and surrogate endpoints: preferred definitions and conceptual framework. *Clinical pharmacology and therapeutics* **69**, 89-95, doi:10.1067/mcp.2001.113989 (2001).

92   Albertsen, P. C., Hanley, J. A., Penson, D. F. & Fine, J. Validation of increasing prostate specific antigen as a predictor of prostate cancer death after treatment of localized prostate cancer with surgery or radiation. *The Journal of urology* **171**, 2221-2225 (2004).

93   Crawford, D. C. *et al.* Genetic variation is associated with C-reactive protein levels in the Third National Health and Nutrition Examination Survey. *Circulation* **114**, 2458-2465, doi:10.1161/CIRCULATIONAHA.106.615740 (2006).

94   Jacobs, J. M. *et al.* Utilizing human blood plasma for proteomic biomarker discovery. *Journal of proteome research* **4**, 1073-1085, doi:10.1021/pr0500657 (2005).

95   Andersson, M. *et al.* Cerebrospinal fluid in the diagnosis of multiple sclerosis: a consensus report. *Journal of neurology, neurosurgery, and psychiatry* **57**, 897-902 (1994).

96   Ahrens, C. H., Brunner, E., Qeli, E., Basler, K. & Aebersold, R. Generating and navigating proteome maps using mass spectro-metry. *Nature reviews. Molecular cell biology* **11**, 789-801, doi:10.1038/nrm2973 (2010).

97   Bantscheff, M., Schirle, M., Sweetman, G., Rick, J. & Kuster, B. Quantitative mass spectrometry in proteomics: a critical review. *Analytical and bioanalytical chemistry* **389**, 1017-1031, doi:10.1007/s00216-007-1486-6 (2007).

98   Prakash, A. *et al.* Assessing bias in experiment design for large scale mass spectrometry-based quantitative proteomics. *Molecular & cellular proteomics: MCP* **6**, 1741-1748, doi:10.1074/mcp.M600470-MCP200 (2007).

99   Zhu, W., Smith, J. W. & Huang, C. M. Mass spectrometry-based label-free quantitative proteomics. *Journal of biomedicine & biotechnology* **2010**, 840518, doi:10.1155/2010/840518 (2010).

100   Old, W. M. *et al.* Comparison of label-free methods for quantifying human proteins by shotgun proteomics. *Molecular & cellular proteomics: MCP* **4**, 1487-1502, doi:10.1074/mcp.M500084-MCP200 (2005).

101   Liu, F., Rong, Y. P., Zeng, L. C., Zhang, X. & Han, Z. G. Isolation and characterization of a novel human thioredoxin-like gene hTLP19 encoding a secretory protein. *Gene* **315**, 71-78 (2003).

102   Voyksner, R. D. & Lee, H. Investigating the use of an octupole ion guide for ion storage and high-pass mass filtering to improve the quantitative performance of electrospray ion trap mass spectrometry. *Rapid communications in mass spectrometry: RCM* **13**, 1427-1437, doi:10.1002/(SICI)1097-0231(19990730)13:14<1427::AIDRCM662>3.0.CO;2-5 (1999).

103   Florens, L. *et al.* Analyzing chromatin remodeling complexes using shotgun proteomics and normalized spectral abundance factors. *Methods* **40**, 303-311, doi:10.1016/j.ymeth.2006.07.028 (2006).

104   Zybailov, B. *et al.* Statistical analysis of membrane proteome expression changes in Saccharomyces cerevisiae. *Journal of proteome research* **5**, 2339-2347, doi:10.1021/pr060161n (2006).

105   Oda, Y., Huang, K., Cross, F. R., Cowburn, D. & Chait, B. T. Accurate quantitation of protein expression and site-specific phosphorylation. *Proceedings of the National Academy of Sciences of the United States of America* **96**, 6591-6596 (1999).

106   Ong, S. E. *et al.* Stable isotope labeling by amino acids in cell culture, SILAC, as a simple and accurate approach to expression proteomics. *Molecular & cellular proteomics: MCP* **1**, 376-386 (2002).

107   Mirgorodskaya, O. A. *et al.* Quantitation of peptides and proteins by matrix-assisted laser desorption/ionization mass spectrometry using (18)O-labeled internal standards. *Rapid communications in mass spectrometry: RCM* **14**, 1226-1232, doi:10.1002/1097-0231(20000730) 14:14<1226::AID-RCM14>3.0.CO;2-V (2000).

108   Stewart, II, Thomson, T. & Figeys, D. 18O labeling: a tool for proteomics. *Rapid communications in mass spectrometry: RCM* **15**, 2456-2465, doi:10.1002/rcm.525 (2001).

109   Chakraborty, A. & Regnier, F. E. Global internal standard technology for comparative proteomics. *Journal of chromatography. A* **949**, 173-184 (2002).

110   Hsu, J. L., Huang, S. Y., Chow, N. H. & Chen, S. H. Stable-isotope dimethyl labeling for quantitative proteomics. *Analytical chemistry* **75**, 6843-6852, doi:10.1021/ac0348625 (2003).

111   Gygi, S. P. *et al.* Quantitative analysis of complex protein mixtures using isotope-coded affinity tags. *Nature biotechnology* **17**, 994-999, doi:10.1038/13690 (1999).

112   Thompson, A. *et al.* Tandem mass tags: a novel quantification strategy for comparative analysis of complex protein mixtures by MS/MS. *Analytical chemistry* **75**, 1895-1904 (2003).

113   Kuhn, E. *et al.* Quantification of C-reactive protein in the serum of patients with rheumatoid arthritis using multiple reaction monitoring mass spectrometry and 13C-labeled peptide standards. *Proteomics* **4**, 1175-1186, doi:10.1002/pmic.200300670 (2004).

114   Picotti, P., Bodenmiller, B., Mueller, L. N., Domon, B. & Aebersold, R. Full dynamic range proteome analysis of S. cerevisiae by targeted proteomics. *Cell* **138**, 795-806, doi:10.1016/j.cell.2009.05.051 (2009).

115   Wasinger, V. C., Zeng, M. & Yau, Y. Current status and advances in quantitative proteomic mass spectrometry. *International journal of proteomics* **2013**, 180605, doi:10.1155/2013/180605 (2013).

116   Wu, B. *et al.* Comparison of statistical methods for classification of ovarian cancer using mass spectrometry data. *Bioinformatics* **19**, 1636-1643 (2003).

117   Yu, J. K., Zheng, S., Tang, Y. & Li, L. An integrated approach utilizing proteomics and bioinformatics to detect ovarian cancer. *Journal of Zhejiang University. Science. B* **6**, 227-231, doi:10.1631/jzus.2005.B0227 (2005).

118   Pratapa, P. N., Patz, E. F., Jr. & Hartemink, A. J. Finding diagnostic biomarkers in proteomic spectra. *Pacific Symposium on Biocomputing. Pacific Symposium on Biocomputing*, 279-290 (2006).

119   Listgarten, J. & Emili, A. Statistical and computational methods for comparative proteomic profiling using liquid chromatography-tandem mass spectrometry. *Molecular & cellular proteomics: MCP* **4**, 419-434, doi:10.1074/mcp.R500005-MCP200 (2005).

120   Wang, P. *et al.* Normalization regarding non-random missing values in high-throughput mass spectrometry data. *Pacific Symposium on Biocomputing. Pacific Symposium on Biocomputing*, 315-326 (2006).

121   Rajathei, D. M., Preethi, J., Singh, H. K. & Rajan, K. E. Molecular docking of bacosides with tryptophan hydroxylase: a model to understand the bacosides mechanism. *Natural products and bioprospecting* **4**, 251-255, doi:10.1007/s13659-014-0031-5 (2014).

122   Saraswat, D., Nehra, S., Chaudhary, K. & Cvs, S. P. Novel vascular endothelial growth factor blocker improves cellular viability and reduces hypobaric hypoxia-induced vascular leakage and oedema in rat brain. *Clinical and experimental pharmacology & physiology* **42**, 475-484, doi:10.1111/1440-1681.12387 (2015).

123   Julian, C. G. *et al.* Exploratory proteomic analysis of hypobaric hypoxia and acute mountain sickness in humans. *J Appl Physiol (1985)* **116**, 937-944, doi:10.1152/japplphysiol.00362.2013 (2014).

124   Ahmad, Y. & Sharma, N. K. An effective method for the analysis of human plasma proteome using two-dimensional gel electrophoresis. *J Proteomics Bioinform* **2**, 5 (2009).

125   Dahl, B. *et al.* Trauma stimulates the synthesis of Gc-globulin. *Intensive care medicine* **27**, 394-399 (2001).

126   Rahman, I., Biswas, S. K. & Kode, A. Oxidant and antioxidant balance in the airways and airway diseases. *European journal of pharmacology* **533**, 222-239, doi:10.1016/j.ejphar.2005.12.087 (2006).

127   Shau, H., Butterfield, L. H., Chiu, R. & Kim, A. Cloning and sequence analysis of candidate human natural killer-enhancing factor genes. *Immunogenetics* **40**, 129-134 (1994).

128   Sarafian, T. A., Rajper, N., Grigorian, B., Kim, A. & Shau, H. Cellular antioxidant properties of human natural killer enhancing factor B. *Free radical research* **26**, 281-289 (1997).

129   Shau, H. *et al.* Thioredoxin peroxidase (natural killer enhancing factor) regulation of activator protein-1 function in endothelial cells. *Biochemical and biophysical research communications* **249**, 683-686, doi:10.1006/bbrc.1998.9129 (1998).

130   Lee, T. H. *et al.* Peroxiredoxin II is essential for sustaining life span of erythrocytes in mice. *Blood* **101**, 5033-5038, doi:10.1182/blood-2002-08-2548 (2003).

131   Geiben-Lynn, R. *et al.* HIV-1 antiviral activity of recombinant natural killer cell enhancing factors, NKEF-A and NKEF-B, members of the peroxiredoxin family. *The Journal of biological chemistry* **278**, 1569-1574, doi:10.1074/jbc.M209964200 (2003).

132   Rousseau, A. S., Richer, C., Richard, M. J., Favier, A. & Margaritis, I. Plasma glutathione peroxidase activity as a potential indicator of hypoxic stress in breath-hold diving. *Aviation, space, and environmental medicine* **77**, 551-555 (2006).

133   Padhy, G., Sethy, N. K., Ganju, L. & Bhargava, K. Abundance of plasma antioxidant proteins confers tolerance to acute hypobaric hypoxia exposure. *High altitude medicine & biology* **14**, 289-297, doi:10.1089/ham.2012.1095 (2013).

134   Weinshilboum, R. M. *et al.* Sulfation and sulfotransferases 1: Sulfotransferase molecular biology: cDNAs and genes. *FASEB journal: official publication of the Federation of American Societies for Experimental Biology* **11**, 3-14 (1997).

135   Turchi, G., Glatt, H. R., Seidel, A., Puliti, A. & Sbrana, I. Structure-activity relationship in the induction of chromosomal aberrations

and spindle disturbances in Chinese hamster epithelial liver cells by regioisomeric phenanthrene quinones. *Cell biology and toxicology* **13**, 155-165 (1997).

136   Coughtrie, M. W. *et al.* Phenol sulphotransferase SULT1A1 polymorphism: molecular diagnosis and allele frequencies in Caucasian and African populations. *The Biochemical journal* **337 (Pt 1)**, 45-49 (1999).

137   Song, E. J. *et al.* Oxidative modification of nucleoside diphosphate kinase and its identification by matrix-assisted laser desorption/ionization time-of-flight mass spectrometry. *Biochemistry* **39**, 10090-10097 (2000).

138   Eaton, P., Byers, H. L., Leeds, N., Ward, M. A. & Shattock, M. J. Detection, quantitation, purification, and identification of cardiac proteins S-thiolated during ischemia and reperfusion. *The Journal of biological chemistry* **277**, 9806-9811, doi:10.1074/jbc.M111454200 (2002).

139   Ahmad, Y. *et al.* Proteomic identification of novel differentiation plasma protein markers in hypobaric hypoxia-induced rat model. *PloS one* **9**, e98027, doi:10.1371/journal.pone.0098027 (2014).

140   Futcher, B., Latter, G. I., Monardo, P., McLaughlin, C. S. & Garrels, J. I. A sampling of the yeast proteome. *Molecular and cellular biology* **19**, 7357-7368 (1999).

141   Varshavsky, A. The N-end rule: functions, mysteries, uses. *Proceedings of the National Academy of Sciences of the United States of America* **93**, 12142-12149 (1996).

142   Lind, S. E. Innovative medical therapies: between practice and research. *Clinical research* **36**, 546-551 (1988).

143   Speeckaert, M., Huang, G., Delanghe, J. R. & Taes, Y. E. Biological and clinical aspects of the vitamin D binding protein (Gc-globulin) and its polymorphism. *Clinica chimica acta; international journal of clinical chemistry* **372**, 33-42, doi:10.1016/j.cca.2006.03.011 (2006).

144   Li, R. C. *et al.* Heme-hemopexin complex attenuates neuronal cell death and stroke damage. *Journal of cerebral blood flow and metabolism:*

official journal of the International Society of Cerebral Blood Flow and Metabolism **29**, 953-964, doi:10.1038/jcbfm.2009.19 (2009).

145   Congote, L. F., Temmel, N., Sadvakassova, G. & Dobocan, M. C. Comparison of the effects of serpin A1, a recombinant serpin A1-IGF chimera and serpin A1 C-terminal peptide on wound healing. *Peptides* **29**, 39-46, doi:10.1016/j.peptides.2007.10.011 (2008).

146   Cowan, K. N. *et al.* Complete reversal of fatal pulmonary hypertension in rats by a serine elastase inhibitor. *Nature medicine* **6**, 698-702, doi:10.1038/76282 (2000).

147   Bowman, B. H. & Kurosky, A. Haptoglobin: the evolutionary product of duplication, unequal crossing over, and point mutation. *Advances in human genetics* **12**, 189-261, 453-184 (1982).

148   Langlois, M. R. & Delanghe, J. R. Biological and clinical significance of haptoglobin polymorphism in humans. *Clinical chemistry* **42**, 1589-1600 (1996).

149   Haugen, T. H., Hanley, J. M. & Heath, E. C. Haptoglobin. A novel mode of biosynthesis of a liver secretory glycoprotein. *The Journal of biological chemistry* **256**, 1055-1057 (1981).

150   Anderson, L. & Anderson, N. G. High resolution two-dimensional electrophoresis of human plasma proteins. *Proceedings of the National Academy of Sciences of the United States of America* **74**, 5421-5425 (1977).

151   Han, C. *et al.* Serum levels of leptin, insulin, and lipids in relation to breast cancer in china. *Endocrine* **26**, 19-24, doi:10.1385/ ENDO: 26:1:019 (2005).

152   Anantharamaiah, G. M. *et al.* Structural requirements for antioxidative and anti-inflammatory properties of apolipoprotein A-I mimetic peptides. *Journal of lipid research* **48**, 1915-1923, doi: 10.1194/jlr.R700010-JLR200 (2007).

153   Bates, S. R., Tao, J. Q., Collins, H. L., Francone, O. L. & Rothblat, G. H. Pulmonary abnormalities due to ABCA1 deficiency in mice. *American journal of physiology. Lung cellular and molecular physiology* **289**, L980-989, doi:10.1152/ajplung.00234.2005 (2005).

154   Ahmad, Y. *et al.* Identification of haptoglobin and apolipoprotein A-I as biomarkers for high altitude pulmonary edema. *Functional & integrative genomics* **11**, 407-417, doi:10.1007/s10142-011-0234-3 (2011).

155   Sylvester, J. T., Shimoda, L. A., Aaronson, P. I. & Ward, J. P. Hypoxic pulmonary vasoconstriction. *Physiological reviews* **92**, 367-520, doi:10.1152/physrev.00041.2010 (2012).

156   Houston, C. S. Acute pulmonary edema of high altitude. *The New England journal of medicine* **263**, 478-480, doi:10.1056/NEJM196009082631003 (1960).

157   Bull, T. M., Coldren, C. D., Geraci, M. W. & Voelkel, N. F. Gene expression profiling in pulmonary hypertension. *Proceedings of the American Thoracic Society* **4**, 117-120, doi:10.1513/pats.200605-128JG (2007).

158   Henschke, P., Vorum, H., Honore, B. & Rice, G. E. Protein profiling the effects of in vitro hyperoxic exposure on fetal rabbit lung. *Proteomics* **6**, 1957-1962, doi:10.1002/pmic.200500245 (2006).

159   Laudi, S. *et al.* Comparison of lung proteome profiles in two rodent models of pulmonary arterial hypertension. *Proteomics* **7**, 2469-2478, doi:10.1002/pmic.200600848 (2007).

160   Kwapiszewska, G. *et al.* Fhl-1, a new key protein in pulmonary hypertension. *Circulation* **118**, 1183-1194, doi:10.1161/CIRCULATIONAHA.107.761916 (2008).

161   Ostergaard, L. *et al.* Pulmonary pressure reduction attenuates expression of proteins identified by lung proteomic profiling in pulmonary hypertensive rats. *Proteomics* **11**, 4492-4502, doi:10.1002/pmic.201100171 (2011).

162   Olmeda, B. *et al.* Effect of hypoxia on lung gene expression and proteomic profile: insights into the pulmonary surfactant response. *Journal of proteomics* **101**, 179-191, doi:10.1016/j.jprot.2014.02.019 (2014).

163   Ahmad, Y. *et al.* The proteome of Hypobaric Induced Hypoxic Lung: Insights from Temporal Proteomic Profiling for Biomarker Discovery. *Scientific reports* **5**, 10681, doi:10.1038/srep10681 (2015).

164   Paul, S., Gangwar, A., Arya, A., Bhargava, K. & Ahmad, Y. High Altitude Pulmonary Edema: An Update on Omics Data and Redefining Susceptibility. *Journal of Proteomics & Bioinformatics* **8**, 116 (2015).

165   Hellman, K. *et al.* Protein expression patterns in primary carcinoma of the vagina. *British journal of cancer* **91**, 319-326, doi:10.1038/sj.bjc.6601944 (2004).

166   Alaiya, A. A. *et al.* Molecular classification of borderline ovarian tumors using hierarchical cluster analysis of protein expression profiles. *International journal of cancer. Journal international du cancer* **98**, 895-899 (2002).

167   Poon, T. C. *et al.* Comprehensive proteomic profiling identifies serum proteomic signatures for detection of hepatocellular carcinoma and its subtypes. *Clinical chemistry* **49**, 752-760 (2003).

168   Hu, Y., Malone, J. P., Fagan, A. M., Townsend, R. R. & Holtzman, D. M. Comparative proteomic analysis of intra- and interindividual variation in human cerebrospinal fluid. *Molecular & cellular proteomics: MCP* **4**, 2000-2009, doi:10.1074/mcp.M500207-MCP200 (2005).

169   Meunier, B. *et al.* Assessment of hierarchical clustering methodologies for proteomic data mining. *Journal of proteome research* **6**, 358-366, doi:10.1021/pr060343h (2007).

170   Belknap, J. K. Empirical estimates of Bonferroni corrections for use in chromosome mapping studies with the BXD recombinant inbred strains. *Behavior genetics* **22**, 677-684 (1992).

171   Jeffries, N. O. Performance of a genetic algorithm for mass spectrometry proteomics. *BMC bioinformatics* **5**, 180, doi:10.1186/1471-2105-5-180 (2004).

172   Petricoin, E. F., Zoon, K. C., Kohn, E. C., Barrett, J. C. & Liotta, L. A. Clinical proteomics: translating benchside promise into bedside reality. *Nature reviews. Drug discovery* **1**, 683-695, doi:10.1038/nrd891 (2002).

173   Ball, G. *et al.* An integrated approach utilizing artificial neural networks and SELDI mass spectrometry for the classification of

human tumours and rapid identification of potential biomarkers. *Bioinformatics* **18**, 395-404 (2002).

174   Li, J., Zhang, Z., Rosenzweig, J., Wang, Y. Y. & Chan, D. W. Proteomics and bioinformatics approaches for identification of serum biomarkers to detect breast cancer. *Clinical chemistry* **48**, 1296-1304 (2002).

175   Zhang, Z. *et al.* Three biomarkers identified from serum proteomic analysis for the detection of early stage ovarian cancer. *Cancer research* **64**, 5882-5890, doi:10.1158/0008-5472.CAN-04-0746 (2004).